LOS
PALEO

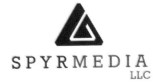

SPYRMEDIA
LLC

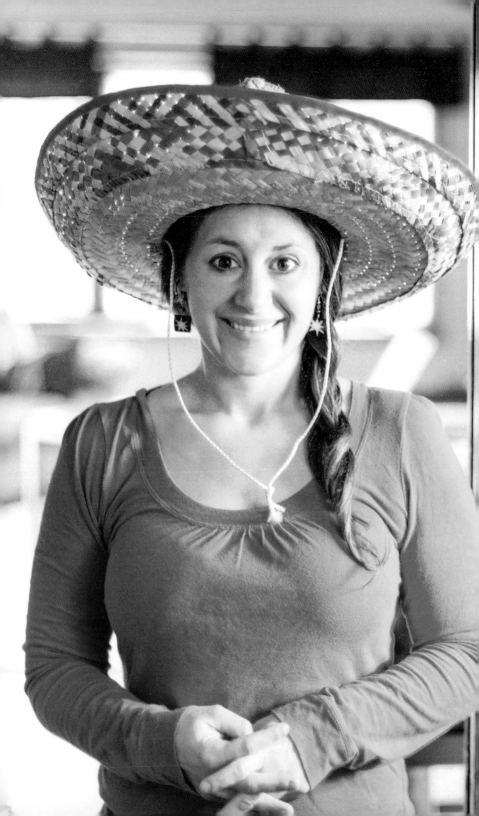

Marla Sarris

LOS
PALEO

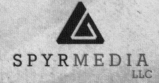

SPYRMEDIA
LLC

□□□□□□□□□□□□□□□□ □□ □□□□□□□□

□□□□□□□□□□©□□□□□ □□□□ □□□□□□□□□□

□ □□□□□□ □ □□□□□□□□□□□□□ □□□ □□□ □□□□□□□ □□□□□□ □□ □□□□□□□□□□□□ □□□ □□□□□□
□□ □□□□□□□□□□□ □□□□ □□□□ □□□□□□□□□□□ □□□ □□□□ □□□ □□□□□ □□□□□□□□ □□□□□□□□□□ □□□ □□□□
□□□□□□□□□□ □□□□□□ □□□ □□□ □□□□□□□ □□□ □ □□□□□□□□□□□□□ □□ □□□□□□□□□□□□□□□
□ □□□ □□ □□□ □□□□□ □□□□□□ □□□□ □□□ □□□□□□ □□□ □□□□□□□□□□

□□□ □ □□ □□□□□□□□□□□□□□□□□□
□□□ □ □□□ □□□ □□□□□□□□□□□□

□ □ □□□□□ □□□□□□□□□□□ □□□ □□□□□□□□□□□ □ □□□□ □□□□□□□□□□□□□ □□ □□□□□
□□ □□□□ □□□□□□ □□□□□□□ □□□□□□□□□□□ □□□□ □□□□□ □□ □□□□ □□□□ □ □□□□□□□□□□
□□□□□□□□□□ □□□ □□□□□□ □□□□ □□ □□□□□□□ □□□□ □ □□□□□□ □□□ □□□□□ □□□ □□
□□ □□□□ □□□□□ □□ □□□ □□ □□□□ □□□ □□□ □□□□□□□

□□□□□□ □□□□ □□□□□ □□ □□□ □□□□□□ □□ □□□□□ □□□ □□□□□□□ □ □□ □□□□□
□ □□□ □□□□ □□□ □□□□ □□□□□□□□□ □□□□□ □ □□ □□□□□
□ □□□□□□□□□□□□□□□□□□□□©□□ □□□□□□ □□□□□□□□ □ □□ □□□□□□

□ □□□□□ □□□□ □

FOREWORD

Recently I was sitting in a coffee shop with Marla and her husband Jeff talking paleo. We somehow stumbled onto the topic of the genres of food that could make eating paleo difficult.

"Mexican", I threw out, hoping to stump her.

"Nah, that's easy", she responded.

"Really?"

"Yeah, it just takes a bit of creativity", as she rattled off a half dozen dish ideas off the top of her head.

We stayed and talked until 3am (thank you 24-hour Chicago coffee shops), and as the coffee shop crowd began to get more and more interesting our initial idea began to take on a life of it's own.

See, when people ask me why I eat a paleo framework, the answer is always the same - it's really simple.

Regardless of the terminology, the paleo framework focuses on eating real food. It doesn't take a genius or a point system to figure it out, and it doesn't take hours and hours of logging food. I've seen people lose weight, reverse diabetes and change their lives with the paleo diet. It just works.

Over the past few years of eating and living paleo, there always seem to be a few constant objections – the most common being that, to an outsider, the paleo diet seems limiting - lean meats, vegetables, fruits, nuts and seeds. While that excuse doesn't always resonate with me (my bachelor self has no issues eating broccoli and chicken night after night), where others see limits, Marla sees an opportunity to practice her creativity in the kitchen - and that's what I love both about her and this book.

Los Paleo takes away any and all excuses you may have to eating paleo.

Even in a food genre that's rife with wheat tortillas, Los Paleo shows you that no matter what dish you're preparing, with a little creative thinking, you can make anything healthier, tastier, and, yes, even paleo.

From a caffeine-fueled, 3am idea in a coffee shop discussion to a tasty (not-to-mention gorgeous) recipe book, Los Paleo is not only the most creative paleo you've seen, but also some of the most delicious.

Put on your bib and get ready to drool. This is Los Paleo.

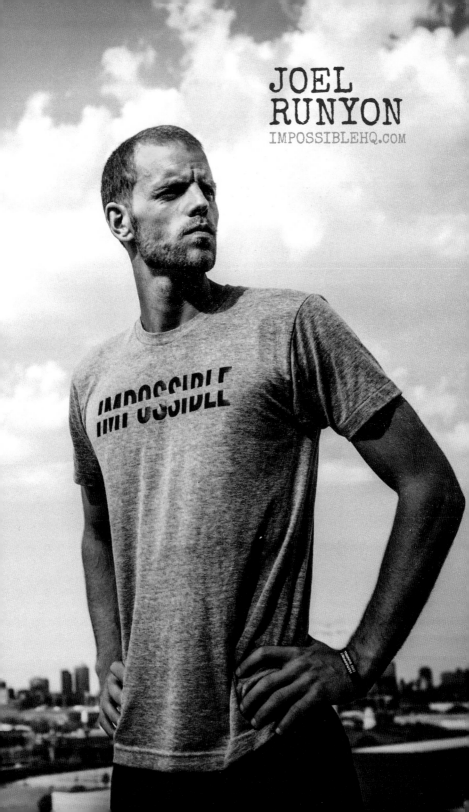

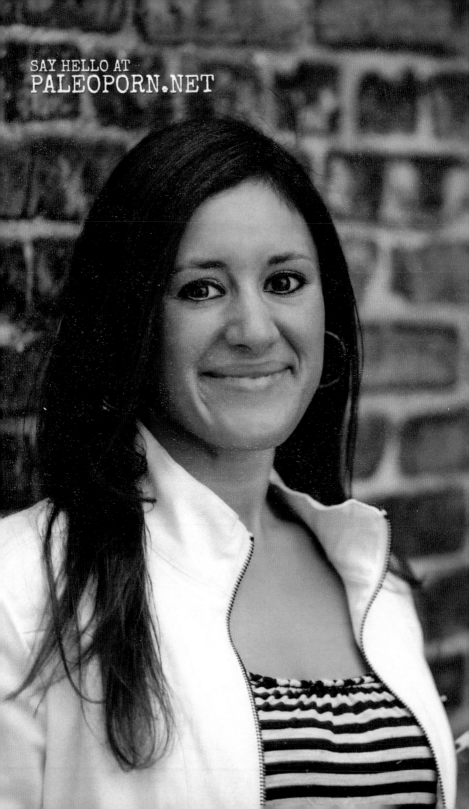

ABOUT MARLA SARRIS

Hey there, I'm Marla Sarris and this book is a little extension of me. In 2010 I quit my job as a high school Algebra teacher and decided to focus on figuring out what I really wanted out of life.

At that time me and my husband Jeff embraced minimalism and paired down to just the necessities. Removing clutter from our lives has been the catalyst that allowed us to discover what truly makes us happy.

After first taking some time out to travel and see the world, I returned home and began spending more time in the kitchen, while Jeff persued expanding his design business (now SPYR Media). Like everyone my experiences in the kitchen didn't start out roses - ask about the "butter the bottom of the pan" incident sometime - but over time, as I learned more and my palate improved I began to really experiment, and to my surprise, receive rave reviews from family and friends. Now I use food as my creative outlet.

We're paleo veterans, living the paleo lifestyle since 2009, but I'm always looking to try something new and rarely cook the same thing twice. Creating in the kitchen makes me happy and I hope that this book will do the same for you and your tastebuds.

Thank you so much for picking up Los Paleo. For more paleo recipes or to chat about fitness come say hi over at my site, PaleoPorn.net.

Enjoy!

SALSA, SAUCES & SNACKS

TOC
MILD · MED · HOT · SWEET

SALADS, SIDES & APPS

ENTREES

DESSERTS & DRINKS

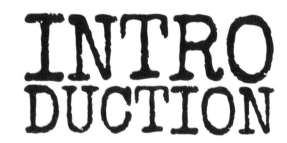

INTRO DUCTION

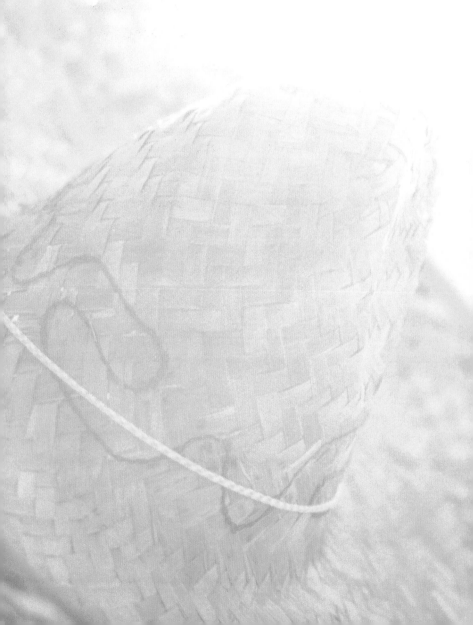

⬛⬛⬛⬛ ⬛⬛⬛⬛⬛ ⬛⬛⬛⬛ ⬛⬛⬛⬛ ⬛⬛⬛⬛⬛ ⬛⬛⬛⬛ ⬛⬛⬛ ⬛⬛ ⬛⬛⬛⬛⬛⬛⬛
⬛⬛⬛⬛⬛ ⬛⬛⬛ ⬛⬛ ⬛⬛⬛⬛⬛⬛ ⬛ ⬛ ⬛⬛⬛⬛⬛ ⬛⬛⬛ ⬛⬛⬛⬛⬛ ⬛⬛ ⬛⬛⬛⬛ ⬛⬛⬛ ⬛⬛⬛
⬛⬛⬛ ⬛⬛ ⬛⬛⬛⬛ ⬛⬛⬛⬛⬛⬛⬛⬛⬛ ⬛⬛ ⬛⬛ ⬛⬛⬛ ⬛⬛⬛⬛ ⬛ ⬛ ⬛ ⬛⬛⬛⬛

⬛ ⬛⬛⬛⬛⬛⬛⬛ ⬛⬛⬛⬛⬛ ⬛⬛ ⬛⬛ ⬛⬛⬛ ⬛⬛⬛⬛⬛ ⬛⬛⬛⬛⬛ ⬛ ⬛⬛⬛⬛ ⬛⬛⬛⬛⬛⬛⬛⬛⬛⬛⬛
⬛⬛⬛⬛⬛ ⬛⬛⬛ ⬛⬛ ⬛⬛ ⬛⬛⬛⬛⬛⬛ ⬛⬛⬛⬛⬛ ⬛⬛ ⬛ ⬛⬛⬛⬛⬛ ⬛⬛⬛ ⬛⬛⬛ ⬛⬛⬛⬛
⬛⬛⬛⬛ ⬛⬛⬛⬛⬛ ⬛⬛ ⬛⬛⬛⬛ ⬛⬛ ⬛⬛ ⬛⬛⬛⬛ ⬛⬛⬛ ⬛⬛ ⬛⬛ ⬛⬛⬛⬛⬛
⬛⬛ ⬛⬛⬛⬛⬛ ⬛⬛⬛ ⬛⬛⬛ ⬛⬛⬛ ⬛⬛⬛ ⬛⬛ ⬛⬛⬛⬛⬛⬛⬛ ⬛⬛⬛⬛ ⬛ ⬛⬛ ⬛⬛⬛⬛⬛
⬛⬛⬛ ⬛⬛⬛⬛⬛ ⬛⬛⬛ ⬛⬛

⬛⬛⬛ ⬛⬛⬛⬛ ⬛⬛⬛ ⬛⬛⬛⬛⬛⬛⬛⬛⬛⬛⬛⬛⬛ ⬛⬛⬛⬛ ⬛⬛⬛⬛⬛⬛⬛⬛ ⬛⬛
immense benefits. Eating real food does evoke a shift in your
⬛⬛⬛⬛⬛⬛⬛⬛ ⬛⬛⬛⬛⬛ ⬛⬛⬛⬛⬛⬛⬛⬛⬛⬛⬛ ⬛⬛⬛⬛ ⬛⬛ ⬛⬛ ⬛⬛ ⬛⬛
⬛⬛⬛⬛⬛⬛⬛ ⬛⬛ ⬛⬛⬛ ⬛⬛⬛ ⬛⬛⬛ ⬛⬛⬛⬛⬛ ⬛⬛⬛⬛⬛ ⬛⬛ ⬛⬛⬛⬛⬛⬛ ⬛⬛ ⬛
⬛⬛⬛⬛⬛ ⬛ ⬛⬛⬛⬛⬛⬛⬛ ⬛⬛⬛⬛⬛⬛⬛ ⬛ ⬛⬛⬛⬛⬛ ⬛ ⬛⬛⬛⬛ ⬛⬛⬛⬛⬛
⬛⬛⬛ ⬛⬛⬛⬛ ⬛⬛⬛⬛⬛⬛ ⬛⬛ ⬛⬛ ⬛⬛⬛⬛⬛ ⬛⬛⬛⬛⬛ ⬛⬛ ⬛⬛⬛⬛⬛
⬛⬛⬛⬛⬛⬛ ⬛⬛⬛⬛⬛⬛⬛⬛⬛⬛ ⬛⬛ ⬛⬛⬛⬛ ⬛⬛⬛⬛⬛

There's just something about the rich flavors and textures and
⬛⬛⬛⬛⬛ ⬛ ⬛ ⬛ ⬛

⬛⬛⬛⬛⬛ ⬛ ⬛⬛⬛⬛⬛ ⬛⬛⬛⬛⬛ ⬛⬛⬛ ⬛⬛ ⬛⬛⬛⬛⬛⬛⬛ ⬛⬛ ⬛⬛⬛ ⬛⬛⬛⬛⬛
⬛⬛⬛⬛⬛⬛⬛ ⬛⬛⬛ ⬛⬛⬛⬛⬛⬛ ⬛⬛ ⬛⬛⬛⬛⬛ ⬛⬛⬛⬛⬛⬛⬛⬛⬛⬛⬛⬛⬛ ⬛⬛⬛
⬛⬛⬛⬛ ⬛⬛⬛⬛ ⬛⬛ ⬛⬛⬛⬛⬛⬛⬛⬛ ⬛⬛⬛ ⬛⬛⬛ ⬛⬛ ⬛⬛⬛⬛⬛ ⬛⬛⬛⬛
⬛⬛⬛⬛⬛ ⬛⬛⬛ ⬛ ⬛⬛⬛⬛⬛⬛⬛ ⬛ ⬛⬛⬛⬛⬛⬛ ⬛ ⬛⬛⬛⬛ ⬛⬛⬛ ⬛⬛⬛⬛⬛⬛
Mexican food without all the corn, beans and flour tortillas?

Well shortly after finishing ⬛⬛⬛⬛ ⬛⬛ ⬛⬛ ⬛⬛⬛⬛⬛⬛⬛⬛⬛⬛ ⬛⬛ ⬛⬛⬛⬛
⬛⬛⬛⬛⬛ ⬛⬛ ⬛⬛⬛ ⬛⬛ ⬛⬛ ⬛⬛⬛⬛⬛ ⬛⬛⬛ ⬛⬛ ⬛⬛⬛⬛⬛⬛⬛⬛⬛ ⬛⬛⬛⬛⬛⬛ ⬛
⬛ ⬛⬛⬛⬛⬛⬛ ⬛⬛ ⬛⬛⬛⬛⬛⬛ ⬛⬛⬛ ⬛⬛⬛⬛⬛ ⬛⬛⬛⬛ ⬛⬛⬛ ⬛⬛⬛ ⬛⬛
⬛ ⬛⬛⬛ ⬛⬛ ⬛⬛ ⬛⬛⬛⬛⬛ ⬛⬛⬛ ⬛⬛⬛ ⬛⬛⬛⬛⬛

⬛⬛⬛⬛ ⬛⬛ ⬛⬛⬛⬛⬛ ⬛⬛⬛ ⬛⬛⬛⬛⬛⬛⬛ ⬛⬛⬛ ⬛⬛⬛⬛⬛⬛ ⬛⬛ ⬛⬛⬛⬛ ⬛⬛⬛
⬛⬛⬛⬛⬛ ⬛⬛ ⬛⬛⬛⬛⬛ ⬛⬛⬛⬛⬛ ⬛⬛ ⬛⬛⬛⬛ ⬛⬛⬛ ⬛⬛⬛⬛ ⬛⬛⬛⬛⬛ ⬛⬛

⬛ ⬛⬛⬛ ⬛⬛⬛⬛

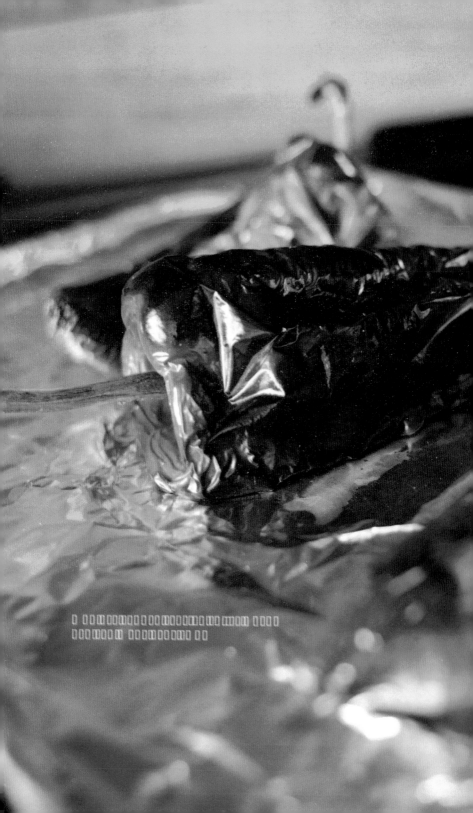

Roasted Green Chiles

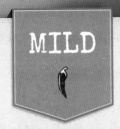

INGREDIENTS (SERVES 6)

3 Cubanelle or Poblano peppers

DIRECTIONS

01 Lay the chiles on a rimmed baking sheet and char under a broiler for 5 minutes. Rotate and roast for another 5-7 minutes. Continue roasting until skins on all sides are semi-charred, brown or loose. This should take 3-5 minutes. (This process can also be achieved on a grill or over an open flame on a gas-stove.)

02 Transfer chiles to a 1 gallon zip lock bag or bowl covered with a dishtowel or tin foil. This will steam the chiles, making it easier to remove the skins.

03 After 10 minutes, or once the chiles are ready to handle with your hands, peel the skins away from the meat of the chiles. Note: Roasted chiles tear easily, so be careful when preparing.

04 Use for Baked Chile Relleno (pg. 81), as an ingredient in salsa or chop & top tacos or salad.

Enjoy! :)

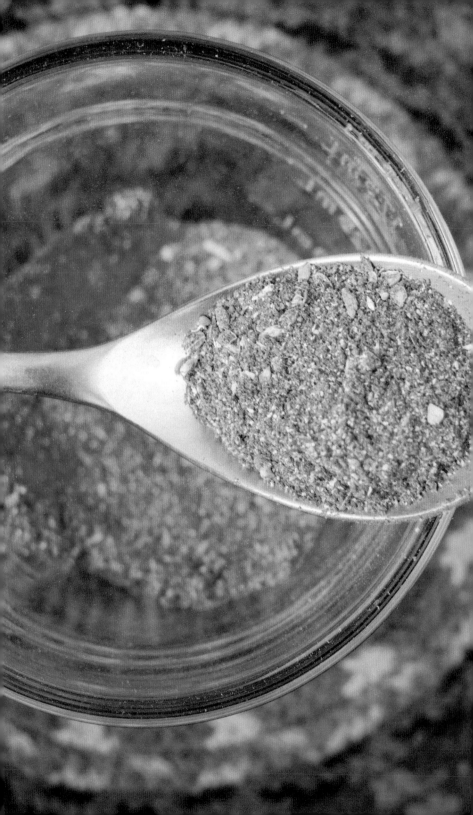

Chili Powder

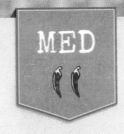

INGREDIENTS (MAKES 1/4 CUP)

- 1 teaspoon paprika
- 1 teaspoon cumin
- 1 1/2 teaspoon cayenne pepper
- 1 teaspoon garlic powder
- 1/8 teaspoon turmeric
- 1/4 teaspoon cinnamon
- 1/4 teaspoon cocoa powder
- 1/8 teaspoon nutmeg
- 1/8 teaspoon ginger

DIRECTIONS

01 Combine paprika, cumin, cayenne pepper, garlic powder, turmeric, cinnamon, cocoa powder, nutmeg and ginger in a small airtight container.

02 Seal and store in a dry, dark place.

03 Use as a taco seasoning for ground beef or bison, to season Dry Rubbed Ribs (pg. 67) or anywhere you would use chili powder.

Enjoy! :)

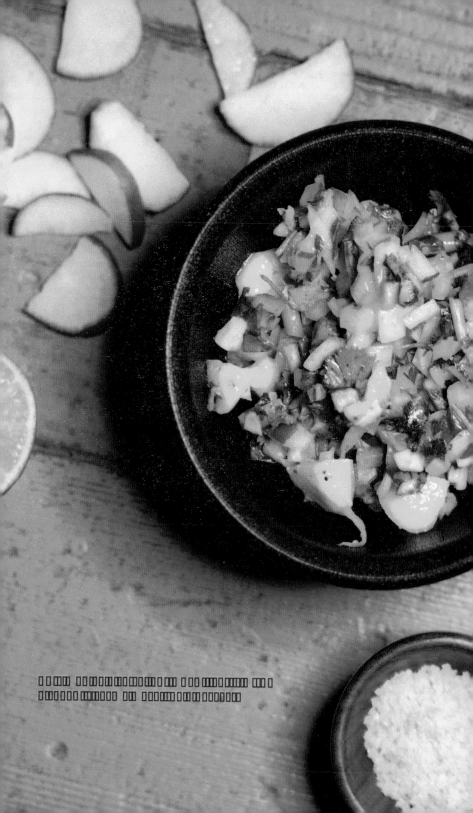

Mango Salsa

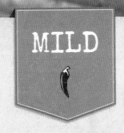

INGREDIENTS (MAKES 1-2 CUPS)

1 golden mango, cubed
1/2 cup red onion, minced
1 1/2 tablespoons olive oil
1/4 cup radish, minced
2 garlic cloves, minced
1/2 cup cilantro, chopped
1/4 teaspoon turmeric
1/2 teaspoon sea salt

DIRECTIONS

01   Add golden mango, red onion, olive oil, radish, garlic cloves, cilantro, turmeric and sea salt to a medium-sized mixing bowl

02   Mix to combine and serve over Fish Tacos with Mango Salsa (pg. 99), with Jicama Chips (pg. 35) or shovel directly into your mouth.

03   Store in an airtight container for 2-4 days - if you can make it that long.

Enjoy! :)

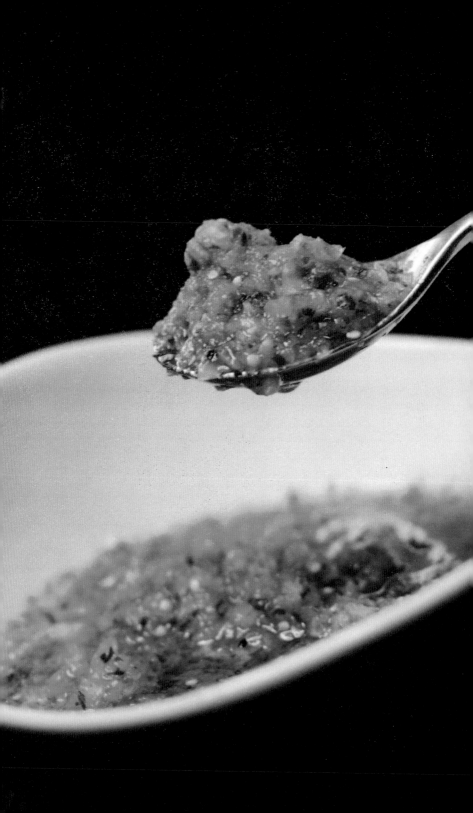

Raw Green Salsa

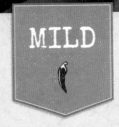

INGREDIENTS (MAKES 3-4 CUPS)

5 tomatillos, husked and chunked

1 small onion

1 bunch cilantro

2 kiwi, peeled

1 jalapeño pepper

2 limes, juiced

pinch of sea salt

DIRECTIONS

01 Add tomatillos, onion, cilantro, kiwi, jalapeño pepper, lime juice and sea salt to a food processor and blend until smooth.

02 Add additional salt, as needed.

03 This salsa can be served a few different ways. Serve over salad, with fresh veggies, Jicama Chips (pg. 35) or to enhance a simply seasoned steak.

Enjoy! :)

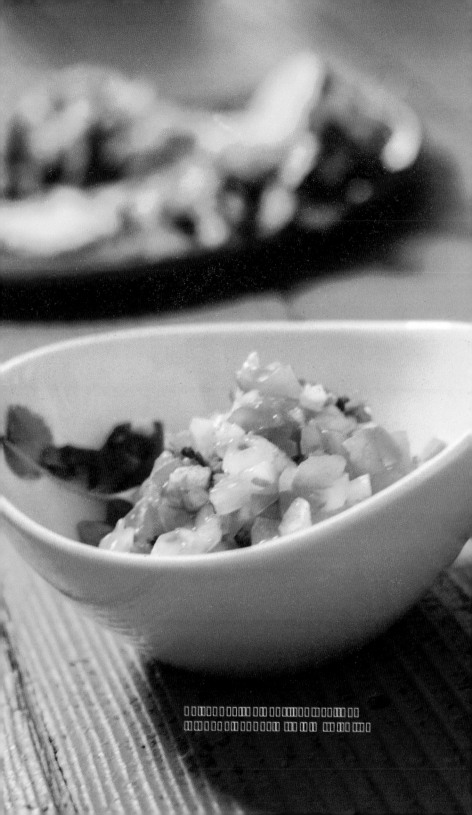

Pico de Gallo

INGREDIENTS (MAKES 2 CUPS)

2 plum tomatoes, chopped
1/2 cup white onion, minced
1 jalapeño pepper, minced
1/2 teaspoon sea salt
fresh cilantro
1 lime, juiced
1 lemon, juiced

DIRECTIONS

01 Combine plum tomatoes, white onion, jalapeño pepper, sea salt, cilantro, lime juice and lemon juice in a medium-sized bowl.

02 Depending on how hot the jalapeño pepper is, you may want to add more sea salt.

03 Serve over Pork Belly Tacos (pg. 79) or scrambled eggs.

Enjoy! :)

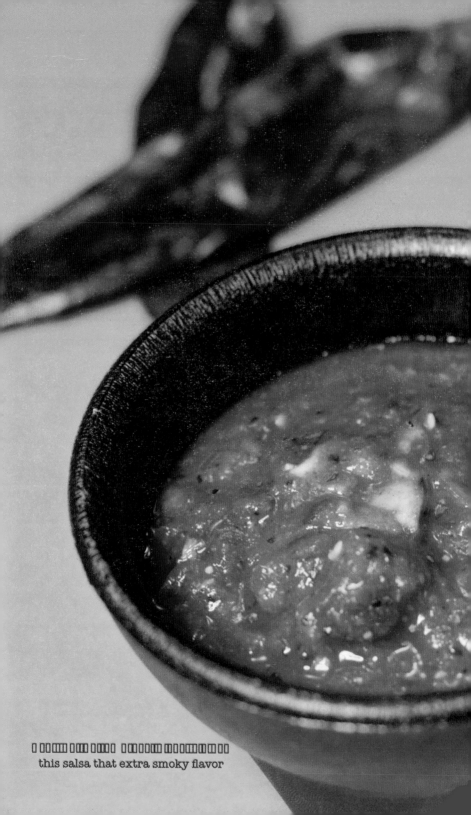

this salsa that extra smoky flavor

Salsa Roja

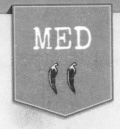
MED

INGREDIENTS (MAKES 2-3 CUPS)

3 guajillo chiles, dried
1lb tomatoes on the vine
8 garlic cloves (skin still on)
1 cup onion, minced
1/2 cup cilantro, chopped
1 serrano chile
1/4 teaspoon ground black pepper
1 teaspoon sea salt
1/4 teaspoon garlic powder

DIRECTIONS

01 Place guajillo chiles in a large bowl and cover with water. Let sit to rehydrate for 15-20 minutes.

02 Rinse tomatoes, remove from the vine and cut each in half.

03 Transfer halved tomatoes to a rimmed baking sheet along with 8 whole cloves of garlic, no need to remove the skins.

04 Place baking sheet under the broiler for 7-10 minutes to blacken the tops of the tomatoes.

05 Add minced onion to a medium-sized mixing bowl and set aside.

06 Remove tomatoes and garlic from the broiler and add to a food processor, reserve 2-3 tomatoes.

07 Remove guajillo chiles from the water, chop off the end, remove seeds and add chiles to the food processor with the tomatoes and garlic. Add cilantro and serrano chile and process until guajillo chiles are finely chopped and salsa is smooth.

08 Transfer mixture from the food processor to the bowl with the onions. Add black pepper, sea salt and garlic powder.

09 Chop reserved tomatoes and add to the bowl. Mix together and serve.

Enjoy! :)

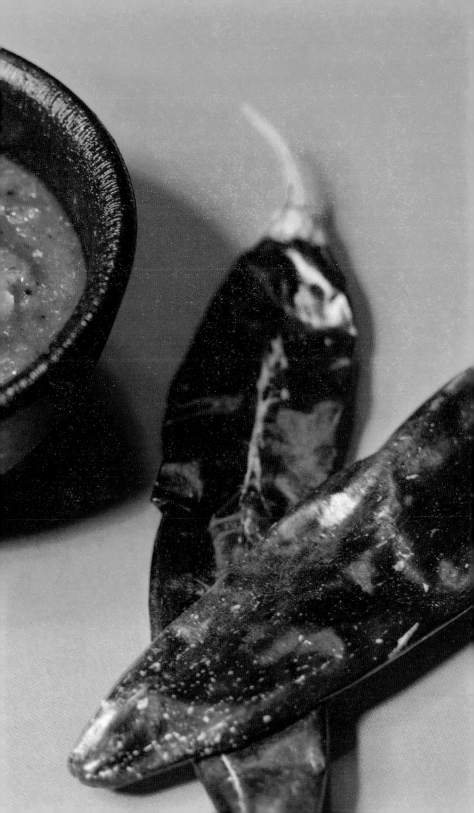

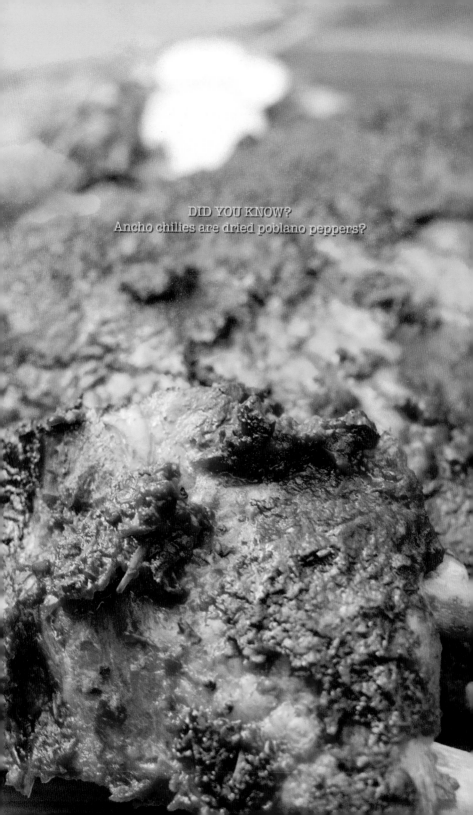

DID YOU KNOW?
Ancho chilies are dried poblano peppers?

Adobo Sauce

INGREDIENTS (MAKES 1 1/2 CUPS)

3 ancho chiles, dried
3 garlic cloves
1 1/2 teaspoons Chili Powder (pg. 17)
2 tablespoons distilled vinegar
2 limes, juiced
1/2 tablespoon raw honey
1/2 cup water

DIRECTIONS

01 Add ancho chiles to a medium-sized bowl and cover with water. Soak chiles until they're soft, approximately 30-60 minutes.

02 Remove ancho chiles from water and chop off the ends. Add chiles (with seeds for extra hot flavor), garlic cloves, Chili Powder (pg. 17), distilled vinegar, lime juice, raw honey and water to a food processor and process until smooth.

03 Use as a marinade for Chile Marinated Shrimp (pg. 101) or Adobo Spiced Ribs (pg. 65). Store in the refrigerator up to five days or in the freezer up to one month.

Enjoy! :)

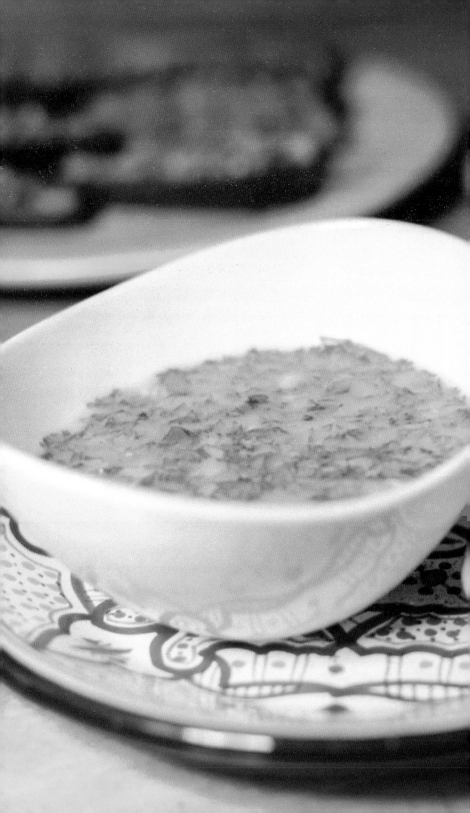

C³: Creamy Coconut Cilantro Dressing

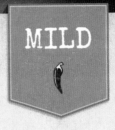

MILD

INGREDIENTS (MAKES 1 CUP)

- 1/2 cup coconut milk
- 1/3 cup cilantro, chopped
- 2 garlic cloves, minced
- 1/4 teaspoon cumin
- 1/2 lime, juiced

DIRECTIONS

01 Add coconut milk, cilantro, garlic cloves, cumin and lime juice to a medium-sized mixing bowl.

02 Stir to combine and serve as a salad dressing or as a dipping sauce for broiled chicken or Chile Marinated Shrimp (pg. 101).

03 Store leftover dressing in an airtight container in the refrigerator for 3-5 days.

Enjoy! :)

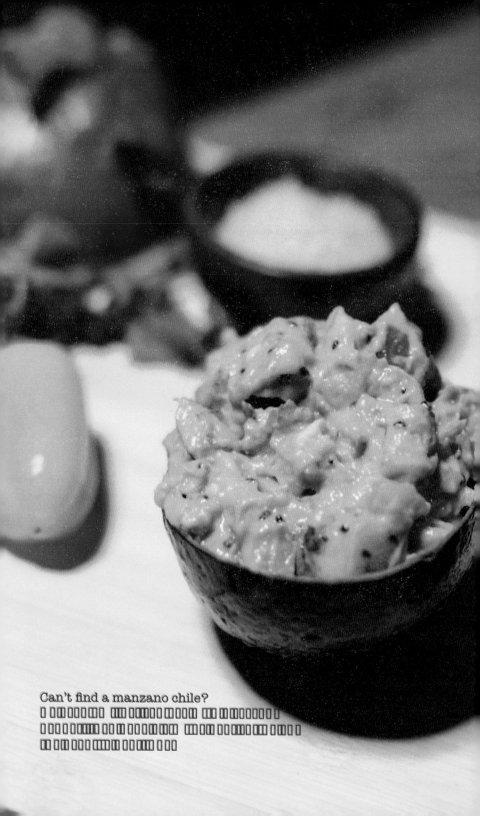

Can't find a manzano chile?
▮ ▮▮▮ ▮▮▮▮▮ ▮▮▮ ▮▮▮▮▮ ▮▮▮▮▮ ▮▮▮ ▮▮ ▮▮▮▮▮▮▮ ▮
▮▮▮▮ ▮▮▮▮▮▮ ▮▮▮ ▮▮ ▮▮▮▮▮▮▮▮ ▮▮▮ ▮▮ ▮▮▮▮ ▮▮ ▮▮▮▮ ▮
▮▮ ▮▮▮ ▮▮▮▮ ▮▮▮▮▮ ▮▮ ▮▮▮▮ ▮▮▮

Dragon Guacamole

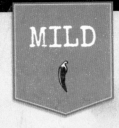

MILD

INGREDIENTS (MAKES 3 CUPS)

3 avocados
1 dragon fruit, chopped
2 green onions, sliced
1 lime, juiced
1/4 cup cilantro, chopped
1 plum tomato, chopped
1 manzano chile, diced*
1 teaspoon sea salt

DIRECTIONS

01 Add avocados to a medium-sized mixing bowl and mash
with a potato masher or a fork. Reserve some chunks, if
you prefer.

02 Add dragon fruit, green onions, lime juice, cilantro,
tomatoe, manzano chile and sea salt to the bowl. Stir to
combine well.

03 Serve with sliced red pepper, whole mini gypsy peppers,
Jicama Chips (pg. 35) or eat with a spoon.

Enjoy! :)

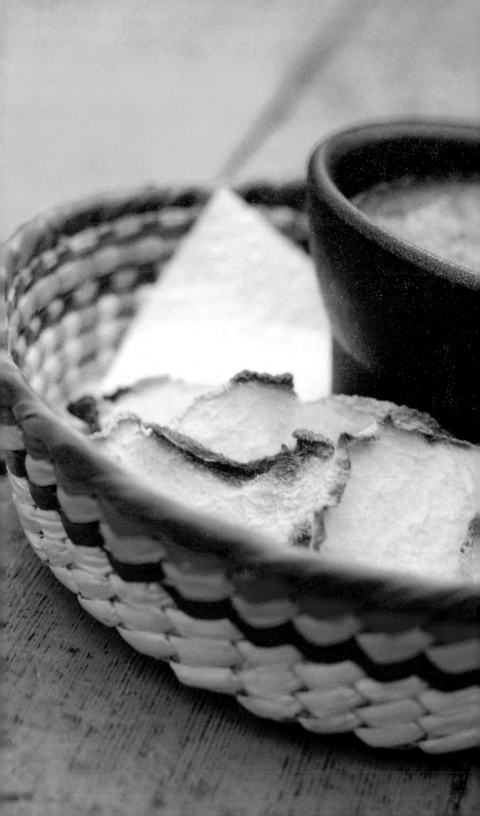

Jicama Chips

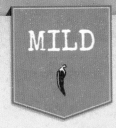
INGREDIENTS (10-12 CHIPS, SERVES 1-2)

1 jicama

DIRECTIONS

01 Preheat the oven to 350 F.

02 Cut ends off of jicama, peel and slice as thin as possible.

03 Elevate chips and lay on a drying rack atop a baking sheet. Bake for 15 minutes, flip and bake for another 15 minutes, or until ends start to curl, but not burn. (Depending on the thickness of the chips, more time may be required.)

04 Remove from the oven and let rest 1-2 minutes. These chips will be crispy around the outer edges with a flimsy texture in the center.

05 Serve with any dipping salsa such as Raw Green Salsa (pg. 21) or Salsa Roja (pg. 25).

Enjoy! :)

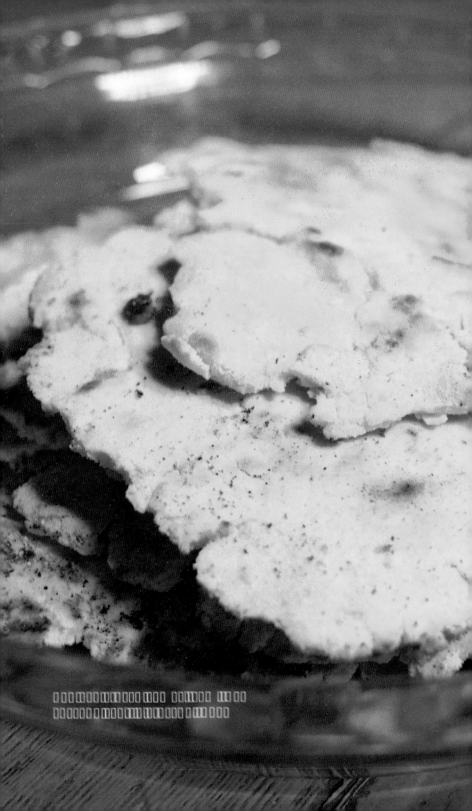

No Corn Tortillas

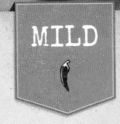

INGREDIENTS (MAKES 8 TORTILLAS)

- 1 cup coconut flour, plus more for rolling
- 1 cup tapioca starch/flour
- 1 teaspoon baking powder
- 1 teaspoon salt
- 4 tablespoons grassfed butter, plus more for frying
- 2 eggs, beaten

DIRECTIONS

01 Combine coconut flour, tapioca flour, baking powder, salt and butter in a large mixing bowl.

02 Add eggs and combine well.

03 Using your hands form 8 balls of dough, transfer to a plate and let rest 10-15 minutes.

04 Prepare to roll the tortillas by spreading a sheet of parchment paper on a cutting board.

05 Roll one of the dough balls in your hands, lightly place it on the cutting board and push down with the palm of your hand. Lightly flour a rolling pin and roll the dough with even pressure in all directions to form a round 1/8" thick tortilla that is 5" in diameter. If the dough cracks as you roll simply re-combine.

06 Heat a griddle or small skillet over medium heat. If using a skillet, melt a little butter and transfer the rolled tortilla to the pan. Cook for 2 minutes on each side. Transfer to a glass container (or between two paper towels on a plate) and keep warm.

07 Repeat steps 5 & 6 until all the tortillas are made.

08 Serve immediately or store in a sealed container for 3-5 days in the refrigerator.

Enjoy! :)

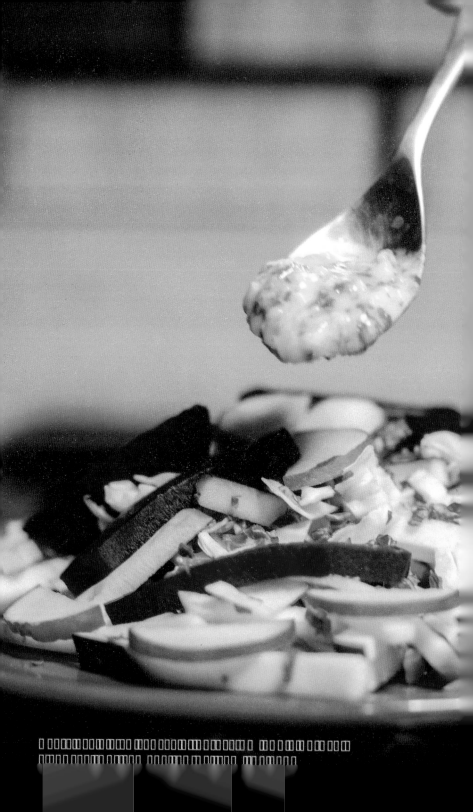

Costa Rican Salad w/Mango Dressing

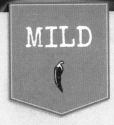

MILD

INGREDIENTS (SERVES 4-6)

- 1 beet, steamed and sliced
- 2 cups green cabbage, shredded
- 1 cup purple cabbage, shredded
- 1 zucchini, ends cut, halved and sliced into matchsticks
- 4-5 radishes, sliced and halved
- 1 teaspoon apple cider vinegar
- 1 lime, juiced
- 3 teaspoons olive oil
- 1 golden mango, pitted
- 1 cup fresh cilantro

DIRECTIONS

01 Bring water to a boil in a double boiler.

02 Peel and slice the beet.

03 Add sliced beet to the double boiler and steam for 15 minutes. Remove from heat and prepare the rest of the salad while the beet cools.

04 Combine shredded green and purple cabbage and zucchini matchsticks in a medium-sized mixing bowl.

05 Plate the cabbage/zucchini mixture. Top with radish halves.

06 Now prepare the dressing. Add vinegar, lime juice, olive oil, mango and cilantro to a food processor and process until no chunks of mango exist.

07 Slice beet into matchsticks and garnish each salad.

08 Drizzle mango-cilantro dressing on top and serve.

Enjoy! :)

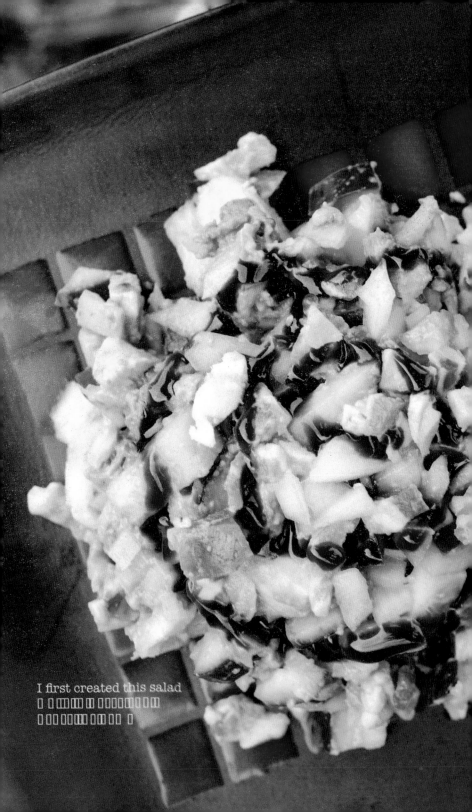

I first created this salad

Chopped Barcelona Salad

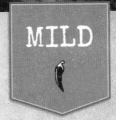

MILD

INGREDIENTS (MAKES 3 CUPS)

- 1 cucumber, diced
- 1 avocado, diced
- 1 cup sweet onion, diced
- 4 oz. pancetta, diced
- 1 teaspoon sea salt
- balsamic vinegar, to taste

DIRECTIONS

01 Dice the cucumber, avocado and onion. Add to a medium-sized mixing bowl.

02 Add pancetta and sea salt and mix to combine.

03 Plate the salad, drizzle balsamic vinegar over the top of each and serve.

Enjoy! :)

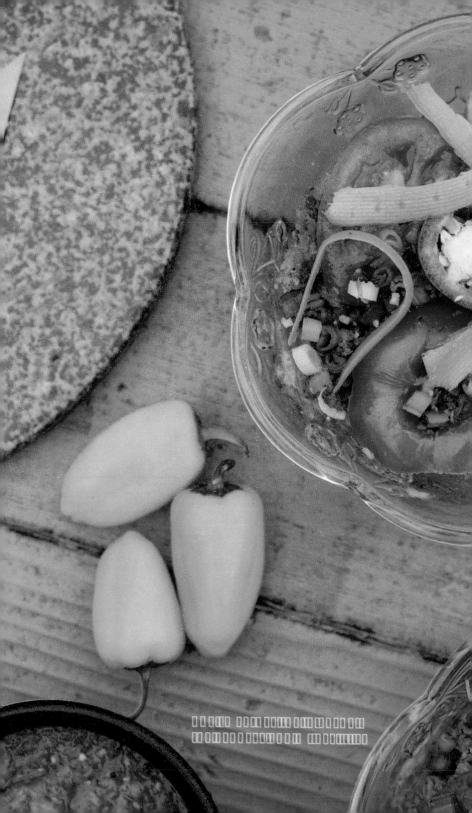

Layered Fiesta Salad

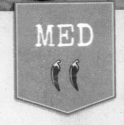

MED

INGREDIENTS (SERVES 3-4)

1 lb grassfed ground beef or bison, browned

1 1/2 teaspoons Chili Powder (pg. 17)

1-2 cups romaine lettuce, sliced

2 tomatoes, sliced

2-3 green onions, sliced

1 jalapeño pepper, sliced

1 carrot, shaved

1-2 limes, halved and juiced

sea salt, to taste

DIRECTIONS

01 Brown the meat, season with Chili Powder (pg. 17), stir to combine well.

02 Once the meat is about done you're ready to build out your layers. Add sliced romaine lettuce to the bottom of serving bowls.

03 Cover the lettuce with a layer of ground beef or bison.

04 Cover the meat with slices of tomato.

05 Sprinkle green onions over tomato.

06 Top with a single slice of jalapeño pepper.

07 Add carrot shavings on top. Season with sea salt.

08 Halve the lime and squeeze juice evenly across the top of all salad bowls.

09 Garnish with a single slice of lime and serve.

Enjoy! :)

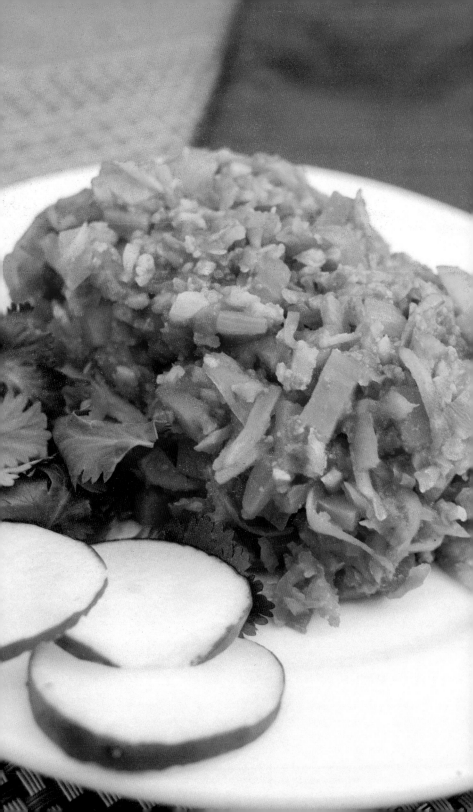

Spanish Rice

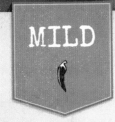

INGREDIENTS (SERVES 2-4)

1 tablespoon grassfed butter
1 cup onion, chopped
2 garlic cloves, minced
1 carrot, finely chopped
3 cups cauliflower, riced
1/2 teaspoon turmeric
1/2 teaspoon sea salt
1/2 cup chicken broth (or water)
1/4 cup tomato paste

DIRECTIONS

01 Melt butter in a large skillet over medium heat.

02 Add onion, garlic and carrot and cook until onions become translucent, around 5 minutes.

03 To rice the cauliflower, use the shred attachment on a food processor. Add the cauliflower rice to the skillet and saute until rice starts to brown. Be sure to stir often. This should take around 5-10 minutes.

04 Add turmeric and sea salt, stir to combine.

05 Reduce heat to medium-low and slowly pour in chicken broth and tomato paste. Stir and combine well.

06 Let the rice mixture warm another 5 minutes.

07 Remove from heat and serve immediately.

Enjoy! :)

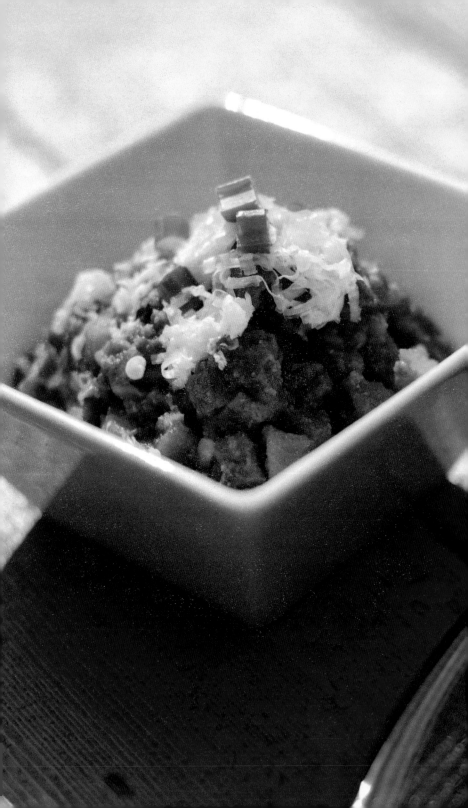

Refried Not Beans

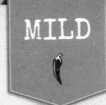

INGREDIENTS (SERVES 4-6)

1 tablespoon grassfed butter (or your choice of fat)

1 large onion, chopped

4 garlic cloves, minced

3 purple potatoes, chopped*

1 banana pepper, chopped

1/2 teaspoon garlic powder

1/2 teaspoon black pepper

1 teaspoon sea salt

1/2 teaspoon cinnamon

1/2 teaspoon cumin

1/2 teaspoon cayenne pepper

shredded cheddar cheese (optional)

green onion, sliced (optional)

DIRECTIONS

01 Melt butter in a large frying pan over medium heat.

02 Add onion and garlic, stir to combine. Cook over medium until onions turn translucent, around 5 minutes.

03 Add purple potatoes, banana pepper, garlic powder, black pepper, sea salt, cinnamon, cumin and cayenne pepper. Stir everything, reduce heat to medium-low and cover.

04 Cook 30-35 minutes, or until potatoes are soft. Occasionally stir the mixture so it doesn't stick.

05 You know the refried beans are done when the potato and onion start to mash together and form a bean texture.

06 Serve warm, topped with shredded cheese (if you desire) and sliced green onion.

Enjoy! :)

* Any sweet potato will do, though purple helps to give that dark color, similar to pinto beans.

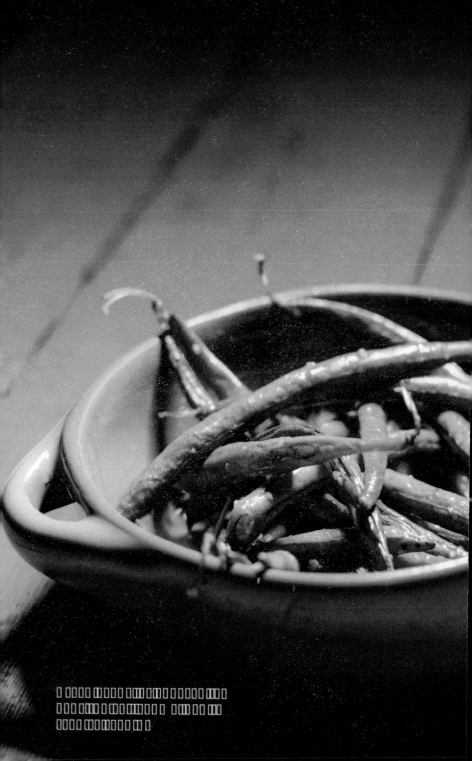

Not the Typical Beans

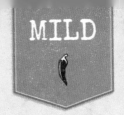

INGREDIENTS (SERVES 2)

10oz green beans, whole
1 1/2 tablespoons olive oil
3 garlic cloves, minced
1/4 teaspoon sea salt
1/4 teaspoon ground chipotle pepper

DIRECTIONS

01 Preheat the oven to 350 F.

02 Rinse green beans and pat dry between two paper towels.

03 Transfer beans to a large mixing bowl.

04 Add olive oil, garlic, sea salt and ground chipotle pepper, mix to combine.

05 Lay the green beans flat on a rimmed baking sheet.

06 Bake for 12-15 minutes.

07 Remove from the oven and serve.

Enjoy! :)

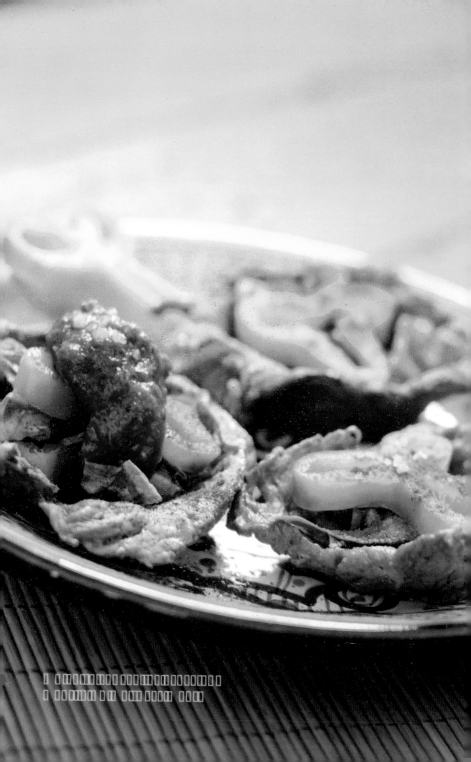

Mini Tender Tostadas

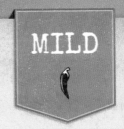
INGREDIENTS (MAKES 12–15)

1lb grassfed bison tenderloin
1 teaspoon coconut oil
1-2 cubanelle peppers, sliced
5-7 romaine lettuce leaves, chopped
paprika, to taste
Salsa Roja (pg. 25)
sea salt, to taste

DIRECTIONS

01 Preheat the oven to 425 F.

02 Place the bison between two slices of parchment paper. With the flat end of a meat tenderizer, pound the bison until thin.

03 Flip a regular muffin tin over and spread coconut oil on the back of each muffin tin.

04 Bake for 5 minutes.

05 Transfer bison cups to a serving platter.

06 Add the following to each cup: romaine lettuce, a slice of cubanelle pepper, a shake of paprika, a scoop of Salsa Roja (pg. 25) and top with a sprinkle of sea salt.

07 If increasing the serving size, store fully prepared tostadas in the fridge. Tostadas can be served cold or warm. Serve as an appetizer, snack or side.

Enjoy! :)

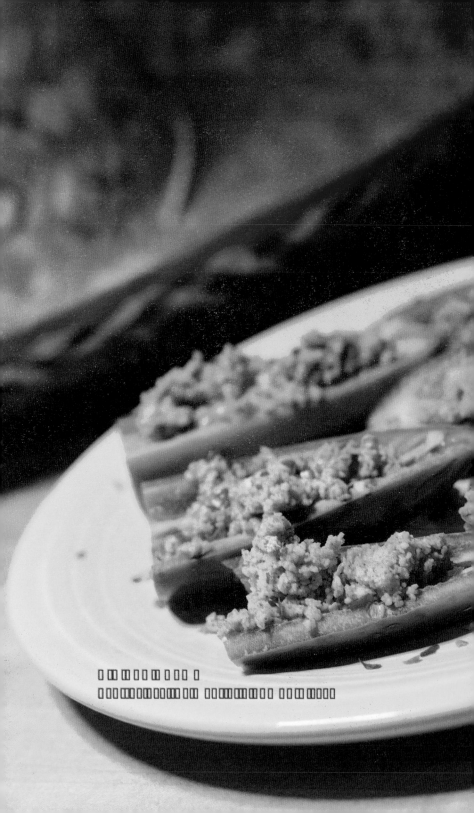

Spicy Nuts in a Pepper Boat

INGREDIENTS (MAKES 16)

1/2 cup whole raw almonds
1/2 cup whole raw cashews
1/2 cup whole raw walnuts
1/4 cup whole raw pepitas
1/2 teaspoon Chili Powder (pg. 17)
1/2 teaspoon paprika
1/2 teaspoon cumin
1/2 teaspoon cayenne pepper
1/4 teaspoon sea salt
2 teaspoons olive oil
2 garlic cloves
8 jalapeño peppers, seeded and halved
red pepper flakes, to taste

DIRECTIONS

01 Add almonds, cashews, walnuts, pepitas, Chili Powder
(pg. 17), paprika, cumin, cayenne pepper, sea salt,
olive oil and garlic cloves to a food processor and blend
until a paste forms.

02 Chop off the tops of the jalapeño peppers, slice in half and
deseed.

03 Add spicy nut paste to each jalapeño pepper.

04 Sprinkle red pepper flakes on top and serve.

Enjoy! :)

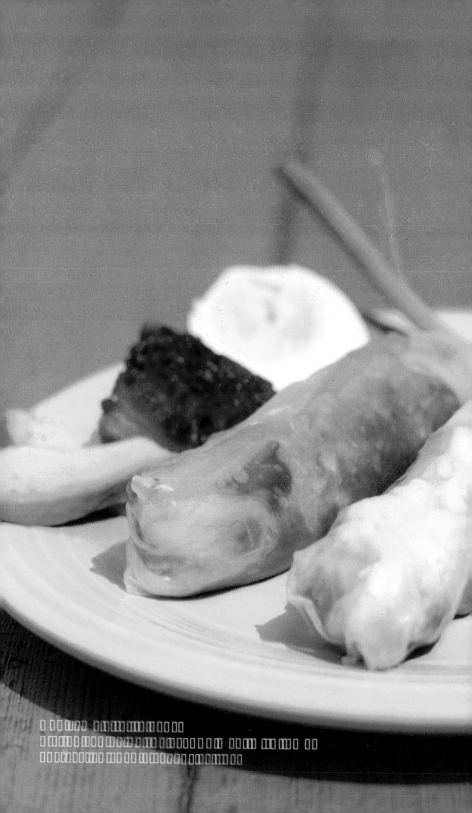

Mini Mexican Burritos

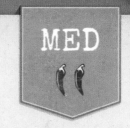

MED

INGREDIENTS (MAKES 12-15)

- 1 tablespoon grassfed butter (or your choice of fat)
- 1 large onion, chopped
- 4 garlic cloves, minced
- 3 purple potatoes, chopped
- 1 banana pepper, chopped
- 1/2 teaspoon garlic powder
- 1/2 teaspoon black pepper
- 1 teaspoon sea salt
- 1/2 teaspoon cinnamon
- 1/2 teaspoon cumin
- 1/2 teaspoon cayenne pepper
- 1lb ground meat (pork, beef, bison, lamb or chicken, etc)*
- 12-15 round spring roll skins
- green onions, sliced
- 2 hard boiled eggs, sliced (optional)
- 1-2 prickly pears (optional)

DIRECTIONS

01 Melt butter in a large frying pan over medium heat.

02 Add onion and garlic, stir to combine. Cook over medium heat until onions turn translucent, around 5 minutes.

03 Add purple potatoes, banana pepper, garlic powder, black pepper, sea salt, cinnamon, cumin and cayenne pepper. Stir, reduce heat to medium-low, cover and cook for 15 minutes.

04 Add ground meat (or be adventurous and use lamb oysters like I did) and stir to combine.

05 Cook 20-30 more minutes, or until potatoes are soft. Occasionally stir the mixture so it doesn't stick.

06 You know the mixture is done when the potato and onion start to mash together with the meat and form a refried bean-like texture.

07 Remove pan from heat, and let's put those burrito's together!

08 Add water to a shallow bowl or rimmed plate that is large enough to accommodate the entire spring roll.

09 Immerse a single spring roll skin in the water, flip over and repeat so both sides are wet and the skin becomes limber.

10 Add spring roll skin to a dry plate, spoon 1 tablespoon of meat and bean mixture onto the end closest to you and start to roll away from you, folding the ends in tight as you roll. When you get halfway lay the sliced green onion in the crease and continue to roll.

11 Continue to repeat step 10 until you've run out of spring roll skins and/or meat and bean mixture.

12 Optionally when you add the sliced green onions you can add hard boiled eggs to the green onions to mellow out the spice. Another option is to add sliced prickly pear to the green onion to sweeten the flavor and compliment the spice. To slice the prickly pear cut off both ends, slice the outside of the pear from top to bottom and peel the outer skin off the pear. Slice the pear in half, remove the seeds from inside and slice the fruit thin enough to add to the green onion. Note: The seeds are edible but unnecessary for this dish.

13 Serve as an appetizer or entree.

Enjoy! :)

* If you're adventurous use offal. I sliced and cubed grassfed lamb oysters (also known as lamb fries or lamb testicles).

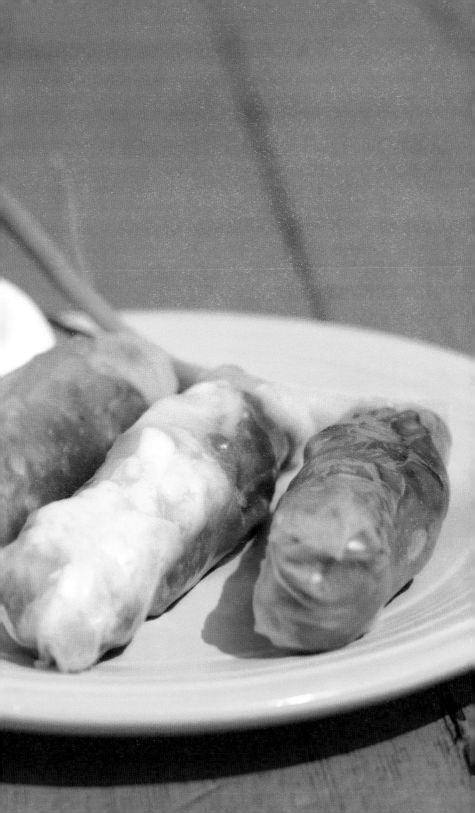

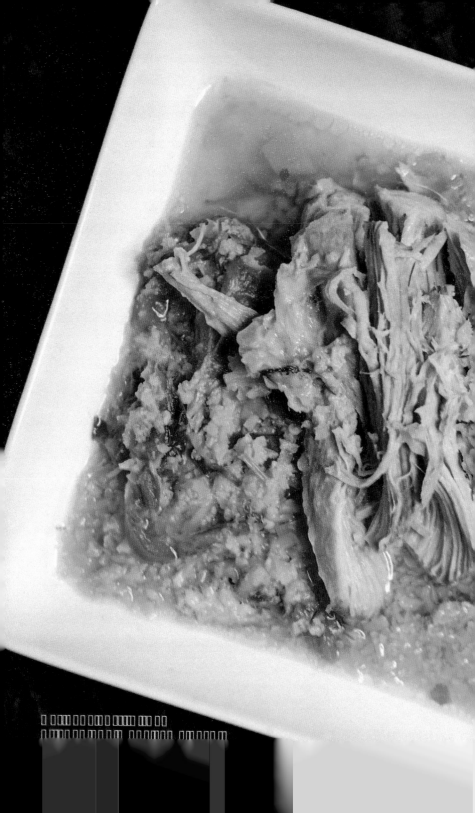

Pork Buttoosk and Riceless Rice

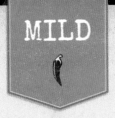

INGREDIENTS (SERVES 8-10)

5-6 lbs pork butt
1 head cauliflower, riced
1 cup cilantro
1 leek, sliced
2 jalapeño peppers, sliced
sea salt, to taste
black pepper, to taste
1/2 cup chicken stock (or water)
2 limes, juiced

DIRECTIONS

01 In a large skillet over medium-high heat brown the pork butt, on all sides.

02 To rice the cauliflower, use the shred attachment on a food processor. Then transfer cauliflower rice to a large crock pot.

03 Add cilantro and leek and combine with the cauliflower in the crock pot.

04 Layer sliced jalapeño peppers on top of cauliflower.

05 Season with a layer of sea salt and black pepper.

06 Add the browned pork butt to the crock pot. You may have to push down to make it fit but it will work.

07 Pour in chicken stock (or water), lime juice and add one of the halved limes in as well.

08 Cook on high for 7-8 hours, or until pork easily falls apart with a fork.

09 Serve with a touch of sea salt.

Enjoy! :)

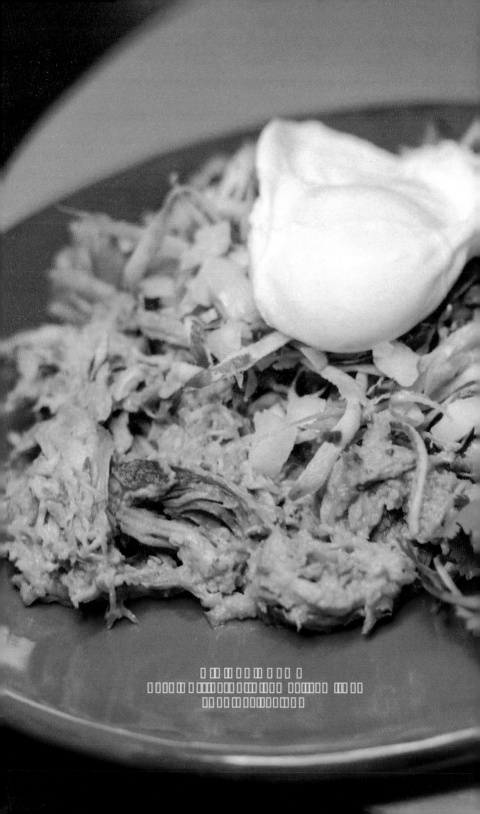

Baconless Pork Breakfast

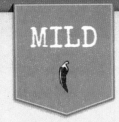

INGREDIENTS (SERVES 2)

2 cups shredded pork butt (pg. 59), cooked
2 eggs, poached (1 per serving)
1/2 cup carrot, shredded
1/2 cup purple cabbage, shredded
1/4 cup white onion, minced
fresh cilantro

DIRECTIONS

01 In a small to medium-sized saucepan warm pork over medium to medium-high heat. Be sure to stir the meat so it doesn't stick to the bottom.

02 Bring water to a boil in a small saucepan to prepare the poached egg. Once brought to a boil, use the back end of a spoon or fork and swirl the water around until a funnel is formed. Crack the egg into the center, reduce heat to medium-low and let the egg cook for 1-2 minutes.

03 While the egg is cooking, plate the warm shredded pork, top with shredded carrots, purple cabbage and minced onion.

04 Remove the poached egg with a slotted spoon and lay on top.

05 Garnish with fresh cilantro and serve.

Enjoy! :)

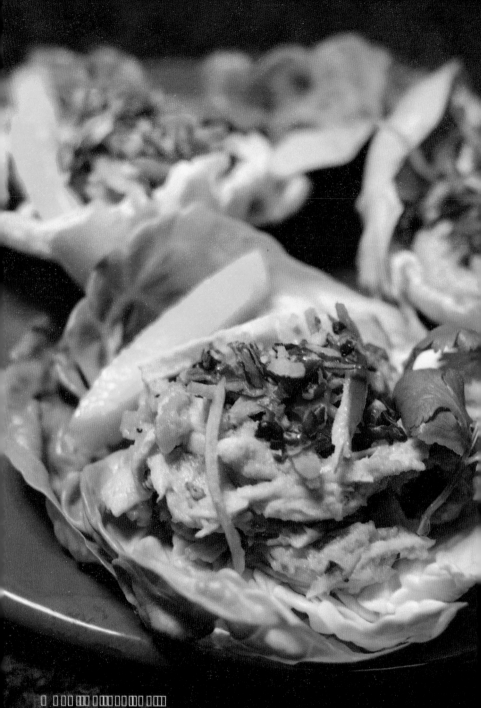

Shred Your Butt Tacos

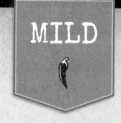
MILD

INGREDIENTS (SERVES 2)

2 cups shredded pork butt (pg. 59), cooked
1 head boston lettuce, leaves washed and separated*
1/2 cup carrot, shredded
1/2 cup purple cabbage, shredded
1 avocado, sliced
1 mango, sliced
fresh cilantro
1 lime, juiced
sea salt, to taste

DIRECTIONS

01 In a small to medium-sized saucepan warm pork over medium to medium-high heat. Be sure to stir so it doesn't stick to the bottom.

02 Carefully tear leaves off the head of boston lettuce, wash and pat dry with a paper towel then set aside.

03 Spoon warmed shredded pork into boston leaves.

04 Top each taco with shredded carrots, shredded purple cabbage, 1-2 slices of avocado, 1-2 slices of mango and finish it off with some fresh cilantro.

05 For a quick hit of citrus, squeeze just a few drops from a lime, add a pinch of sea salt and serve.

Enjoy! :)

* Boston lettuce is also known as butterhead or bibb.

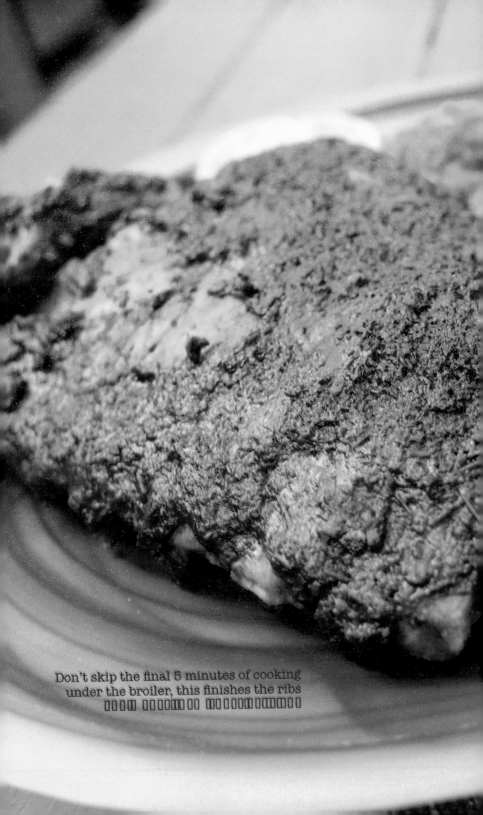

Don't skip the final 5 minutes of cooking
under the broiler, this finishes the ribs

Adobo Spiced Ribs

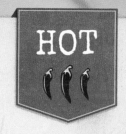

INGREDIENTS (SERVES 2)

1 lb pork baby back loin ribs
sea salt, to taste
black pepper, to taste
1 1/2 cups Adobo Sauce (pg. 29)

DIRECTIONS

01 If frozen, allow ribs to thaw before you begin.

02 Preheat the oven to 350 F.

03 Season the ribs on both sides with sea salt and black pepper.

04 Wrap the ribs in two layers of aluminum foil and bake for 1 1/2 hours.

05 Remove the ribs from the foil and turn the oven to Broil.

06 Baste the Adobo Sauce (pg. 29) on both sides of the ribs and transfer just the ribs (no foil) to the broiler for 5 minutes.

07 Remove from the oven and serve with Spanish Rice (pg. 45).

Enjoy! :)

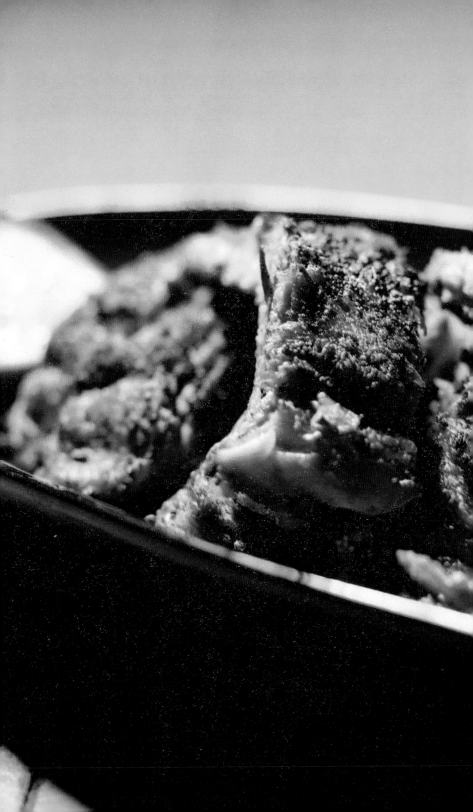

Dry Rubbed Ribs

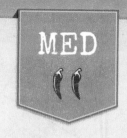

INGREDIENTS (SERVES 2)

1 lb pork baby back loin ribs
2 tablespoons Chili Powder (pg. 17)

DIRECTIONS

01 Thaw the ribs, if frozen.

02 Preheat the oven to 350 F.

03 Rub both sides of the ribs with Chili Powder (pg. 17).

04 Lay ribs on a rimmed baking sheet and bake for 1 1/2 hours.

05 Remove from the oven and serve.

Enjoy! :)

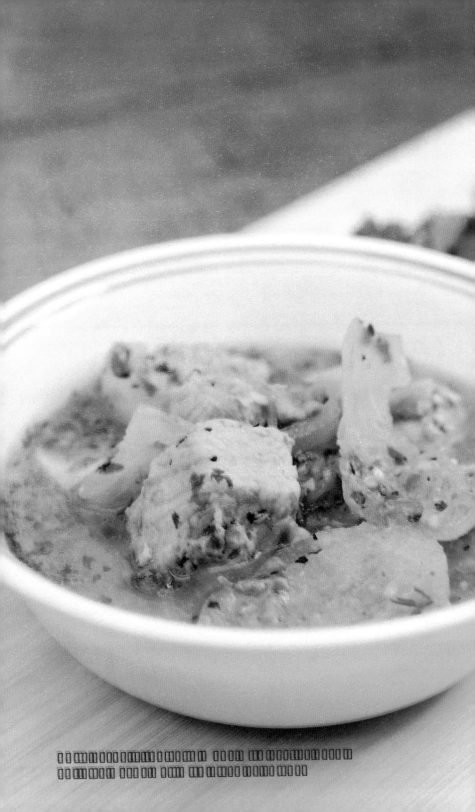

Chile Verde

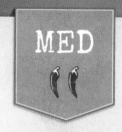
MED

INGREDIENTS (SERVES 6-8)

3 lbs boneless pork shoulder, cubed
sea salt, to taste
coarse ground black pepper, to taste
3/4 - 1 lb tomatillos (about 4-6), husked and halved
8 garlic cloves, skins still on
2 jalapeño peppers, stemmed, seeded and halved
1 Anaheim chile, stemmed, seeded and halved
1 bunch fresh cilantro, plus more for garnish
1 large onion, chopped
2 cups chicken broth

DIRECTIONS

01 Season cubed pork with sea salt and black pepper.

02 Brown pork on all sides in a large skillet over medium
heat. Transfer browned pork to a large crockpot.

03 Husk tomatillos and rinse under water to remove
stickiness on skin, then halve. Add whole garlic cloves
(skins still on), seeded and halved jalapeño and Anaheim
chiles and tomatillo halves to a baking sheet and broil for
8-10 minutes, or until pepper skins turn black.

04 Remove the tray from the broiler. Transfer peppers to a
1 gallon zip lock bag or sealable container to steam for 5
minutes. Let the remaining ingredients rest on the tray
for 5 minutes.

05 Transfer garlic, with skins removed, and tomatillos to a
food processor.

06 Remove chiles from container, remove skins and add
to the food processor. Add cilantro and process until
smooth.

07   Add large chopped onion to pork in crockpot.

08   Pour tomatillo mixture over pork and onion. Mix
     everything in the crockpot.

09   Add chicken broth and cook on high for 3 hours.

10   Serve in a bowl topped with fresh cilantro and a side of
     Spanish Rice (pg. 45).

Enjoy! :)

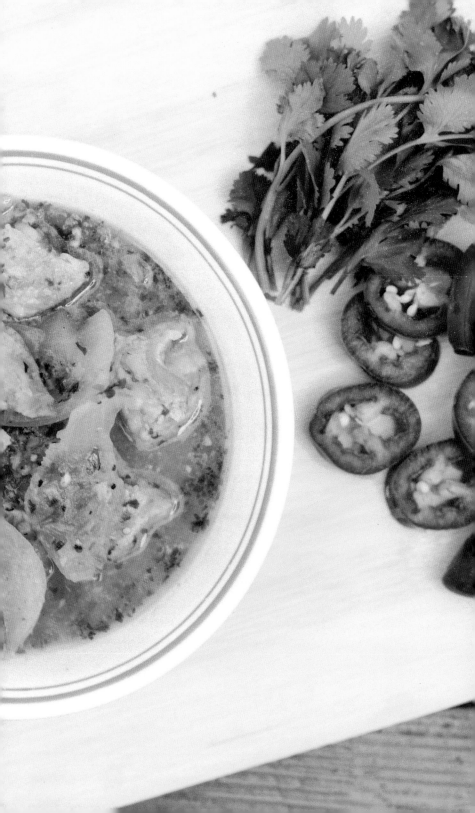

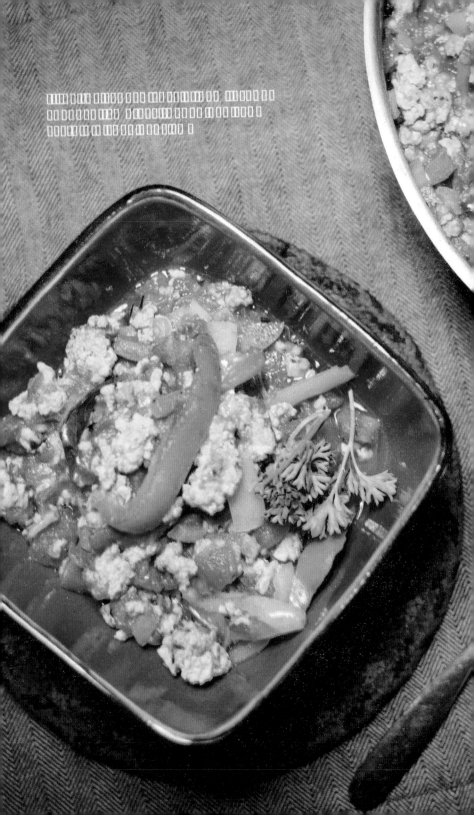

Deconstructed Stuffed Peppers

HOT

INGREDIENTS (SERVES 2)

1lb ground pork
2 garlic cloves, minced
1/2 teaspoon black pepper
1/2 teaspoon sea salt
1 teaspoon garlic powder
1/2 teaspoon onion powder
1/4 teaspoon dried basil
1/4 teaspoon dried oregano
1/4 teaspoon coriander
1/4 teaspoon dried thyme
1/2 large onion, minced (or one small onion)
1 green pepper, thinly sliced
1 banana pepper, thinly sliced
4-6 fresh basil leaves, torn
1 box (26.46oz) chopped tomatoes
fresh parsley (optional)
fresh cilantro (optional)

DIRECTIONS

01 Add the ground pork to a skillet over medium heat. Stir in minced garlic, black pepper, sea salt, garlic powder, onion powder, dried basil, dried oregano, coriander, dried thyme and brown the meat.

02 Stir in onion, green and banana peppers, fresh basil and chopped tomatoes.

03 Bring to a boil, cover and simmer for 15-20 minutes.

04 Pour into a bowl, garnish with fresh parsley or cilantro and serve.

Enjoy! :)

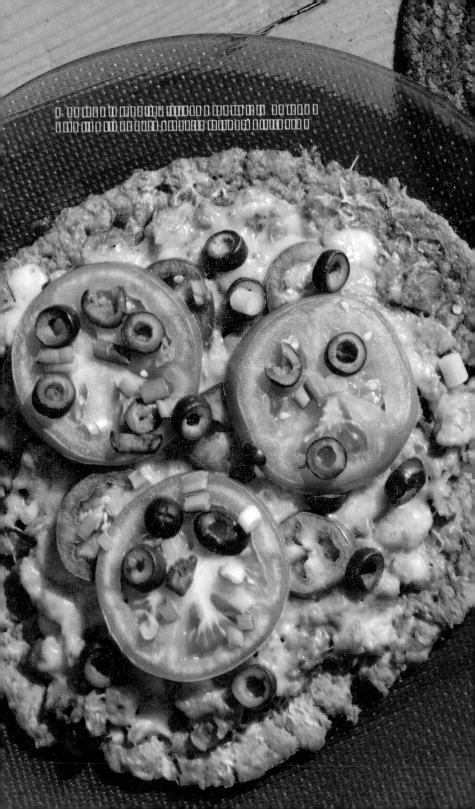

Yo Quiero Pizza

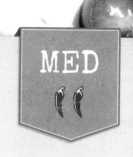

INGREDIENTS (SERVES 3-4)

1 lb ground pork
1/2 tablespoon oregano
1/4 tablespoon sea salt
1 egg
1 1/2 cups Refried Not Beans (pg. 47)
2oz shredded cheddar cheese (optional)*
1 jalapeño pepper, sliced
1 tomato, thinly sliced
1/4 cup black olives, sliced
1 green onion, sliced

*I highly recommend Kerrygold grassfed cheddar cheese

DIRECTIONS

01 Preheat the oven to 375 F.

02 In a medium-sized mixing bowl add ground pork, oregano, sea salt and egg. Using both hands, dig in and blend - don't forget to remove your rings :)

03 Lay a piece of parchment paper across a circular or rectangular rimmed baking sheet. Pour the pork mixture onto the parchment paper and use your hands to flatten the meat as thinly as possible. Once you've done as much as you can with your hands, wrap a wooden rolling pin with parchment paper and roll the pork, avoiding tearing. If you want to go the extra mile and really make it look perfect use a butter knife to trim any excess meat around the edges so the circle or rectangle is how you'd like to present it. Set the excess meat aside to cook and have as a snack. Note: This meat crust will shrink once cooked.

04 Bake pork in the oven for 10 minutes.

05 Remove from the oven. Use a paper towel to pat any excess fat away then flip the pork over, using the parchment paper to help.

06 Bake for another 5-7 minutes.

07 Remove from the oven and let rest 5-10 minutes.

08 Top with a layer of Refried Not Beans (pg. 47), then shred cheddar cheese on top (if desired), layer sliced jalapeño peppers and sliced tomato and top with black olives.

09 Return to the oven for 7-10 more minutes.

10 Take out of the oven, top with sliced green onions and serve.

Enjoy! :)

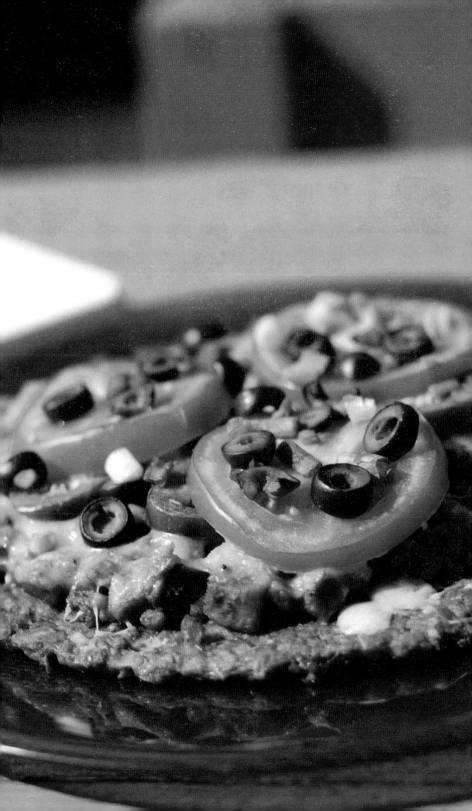

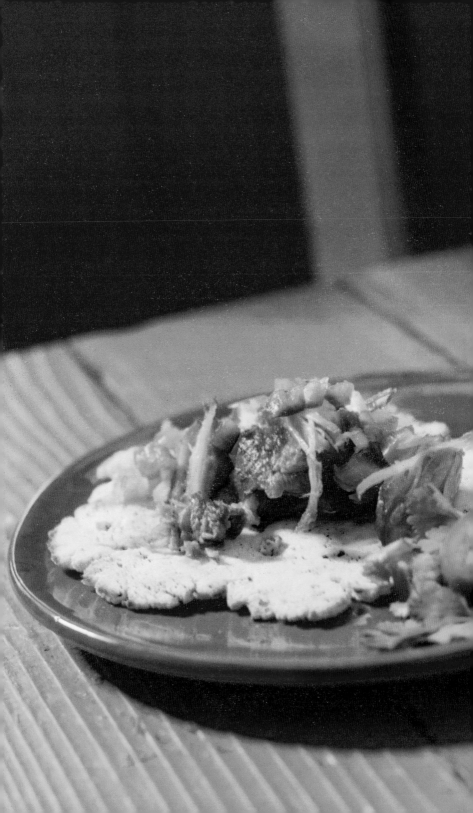

Pork Belly Tacos

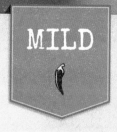

INGREDIENTS (SERVES 2-4)

2-3 lbs pork belly
1-2 teaspoons of sea salt
No Corn Tortillas (pg. 37)
Pico de Gallo (pg. 23)
fresh cilantro
1 lime, quartered

DIRECTIONS

01　Add pork belly to a 1 gallon zip lock bag or large glass bowl and add sea salt. Blend the salt and pork belly, cover and refrigerate for 24-48 hours.

02　Preheat oven to 350 F.

03　Rinse salt off pork belly and transfer to a drying rack over a rimmed baking sheet. Elevating the pork belly will allow the heat to circulate and the rimmed baking sheet will collect all the drippings.

04　Bake for 1 hour at 350 F then drop the heat to 300 F for the second hour of cooking.

05　Carefully remove the pork belly from the oven, so you don't spill the drippings and let it rest for 20-30 minutes.

06　When pork belly is cooled, tear the meat from the bone and fat, shred and set aside.

07　Add pork belly to No Corn Tortillas (pg. 37) and top with Pico de Gallo (pg. 23). Garnish with a side of cilantro and a lime wedge.

Enjoy! :)

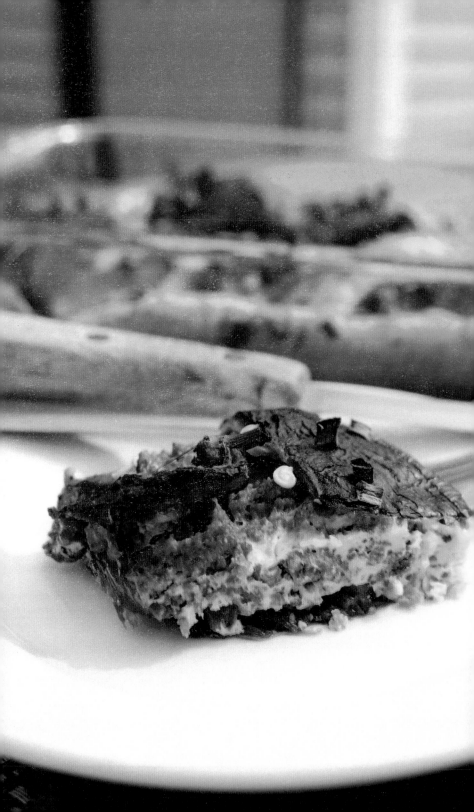

Baked Chile Relleno

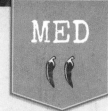

MED

INGREDIENTS (SERVES 6-8)

6 poblano peppers
1 lb grassfed ground bison
1/2 teaspoon paprika
1 teaspoon coriander
1 1/2 teaspoons sea salt
1 teaspoon black pepper
1 teaspoon cayenne pepper
10 extra large eggs
1/2 teaspoon arrowroot starch
3 bunches green onion, sliced

DIRECTIONS

01 Set your oven to Broil. Place all 6 poblano peppers on a foil lined baking tray and broil 8 minutes on one side, flip, and broil 5 minutes on the other side.

02 While the peppers are in the oven brown the bison in a large skillet over medium heat.

03 After five minutes, add the paprika, coriander, 1/2 teaspoon of sea salt, 1/2 teaspoon of black pepper and cayenne pepper to the bison. Stir to combine well. Bison will cook faster than ground beef (if you make a substitution, keep your eye on the meat as you move forward with the rest of the recipe).

04 When the peppers are done, remove them from the oven and transfer them to a glass dish with a lid or a sealed 1 gallon zip lock bag. Let them sit for 10-15 minutes.

05 Preheat the oven to 375 F

06 While you're waiting for the peppers to do their thing, crack 10 eggs into a large mixing bowl. Add 1/2 teaspoon

black pepper, 1 teaspoon sea salt and arrowroot and whisk until combined.

07   Slice green onions and set aside.

08   Peel the outer skins off the peppers. Cut off the top and remove the seeds.

09   Gently stuff the bison mixture into each pepper and transfer each stuffed pepper to a 9x13 glass baking dish. Continue this until all peppers are stuffed.

10   Pour the egg mixture between the gaps of the peppers in the dish.

11   Top the egg and pepper dish with the sliced green onions.

12   Bake for 35 minutes or until a toothpick comes out clean when inserted into the egg.

13   Remove from oven, let sit 5 minutes, cut and serve.

Enjoy! :)

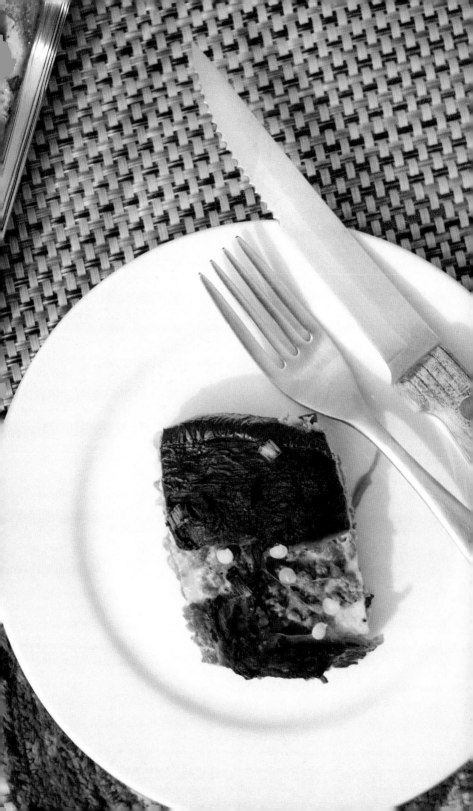

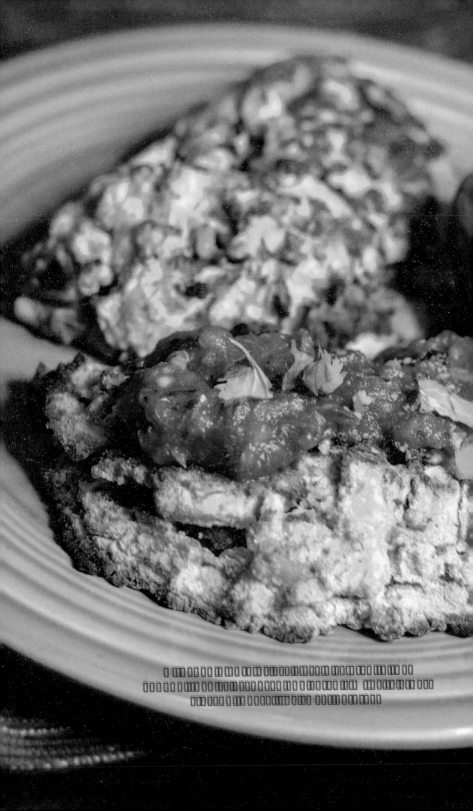

Plantain Empanadas

INGREDIENTS (SERVES 3-4)

1-1 1/2 lbs plantains
1/2 teaspoon raw honey
1/2 lb grassfed ground bison
sea salt (optional)
cinnamon (optional)

DIRECTIONS

01 Preheat oven to 400 F.

02 Add whole plantains to a deep pot covered in water. Boil for 15-30 minutes, or until plantains start to get soft.

03 Remove plantains from boiling water and let sit 5 minutes or until ready to handle.

04 Slice the ends off the plantains and slice down the center of the plantain. Transfer the plantains into a large mixing bowl. Repeat this process for all the boiled plantains.

05 Add raw honey to the plantains.

06 Using a potato masher, smash all the plantains into smaller chunks and make a smooth mixture.

07 Scoop a spoonful of the mixture into your hands. On a cutting board lined with parchment paper, roll out or flatten mixture into a circle.

08 Add a teaspoon of ground bison to half of the circle. Fold the other half over the meat and press to close.

09 Repeat the process and transfer empanadas to a rimmed baking sheet.

10 Season each with sea salt or cinnamon and more raw honey, or bake as is.

11 Bake for 5-10 minutes.

12 Transfer to the broiler for an additional 2-4 minutes.

13 Serve warm or cold, topped with Salsa Roja (pg. 25).

Enjoy! :)

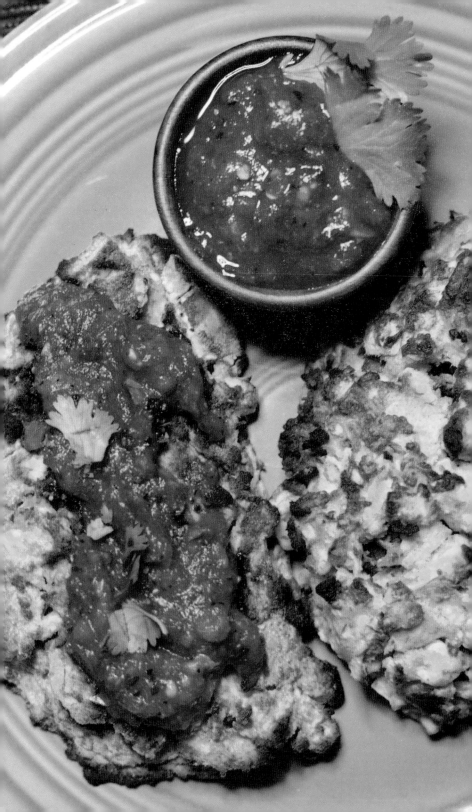

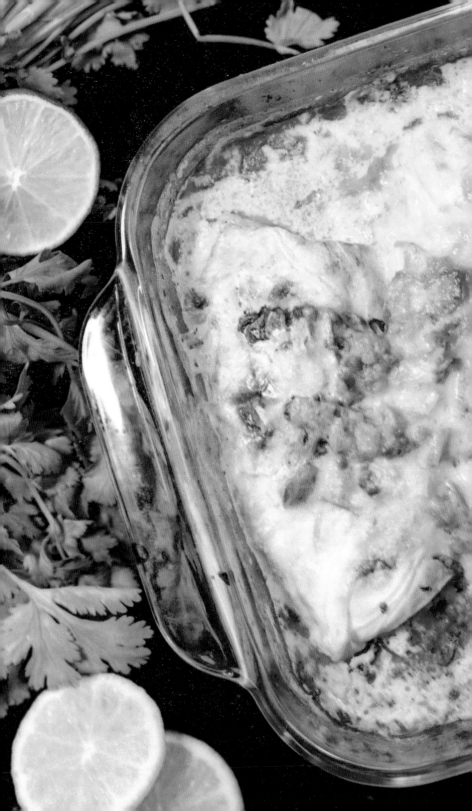

Spicy Chorizo Enchiladas

HOT

INGREDIENTS (SERVES 6)

8-10 green cabbage, leaves
1 cup chicken broth
1 cup coconut milk
2 jalapeño peppers, stems removed and chopped
sea salt, to taste
ground black pepper, to taste
12-16oz chorizo
1 cup fresh cilantro, chopped
1 cup cauliflower, riced
grassfed white cheddar cheese, shredded (optional)
avocado, sliced (optional)
salsa (optional)
limes (optional)

DIRECTIONS

01   Preheat the oven to 350 F.

02   Bring a large pot of water to a boil. Gently peel the leaves
off the head of cabbage making sure they don't tear.
Immerse the cabbage leaves into the pot of boiling water
for 1 minute. Using tongs remove the leaves and set on a
paper towel to dry.

03   Now, let's prepare the enchilada sauce. Add the chicken
broth to a small saucepan over medium heat and bring to
a boil. Lower the heat on the small saucepan and mix in
coconut milk and chopped jalapeño peppers. Stir in the
sea salt and black pepper and let simmer 3-5 minutes.
Remove from heat.

04   Meanwhile, brown the chorizo in a small frying pan over
medium heat, 7-10 minutes.

05 Add chorizo, cilantro and cauliflower rice to a medium-sized mixing bowl. Use a fork to combine.

06 Pour half of the enchilada sauce into a large glass baking dish.

07 Spoon 1-2 teaspoons of chorizo mixture into each cabbage leaf, roll up and add to baking dish. Add remaining chorizo mixture to the dish, between the cabbage enchiladas.

08 Pour remaining enchilada sauce over the top of each enchilada.

09 Top with shredded cheese, if desired.

10 Bake for 25-30 minutes.

11 Serve with sliced avocado, mild salsa, more fresh cilantro and/or a lime wedge to tame the flame.

Enjoy! :)

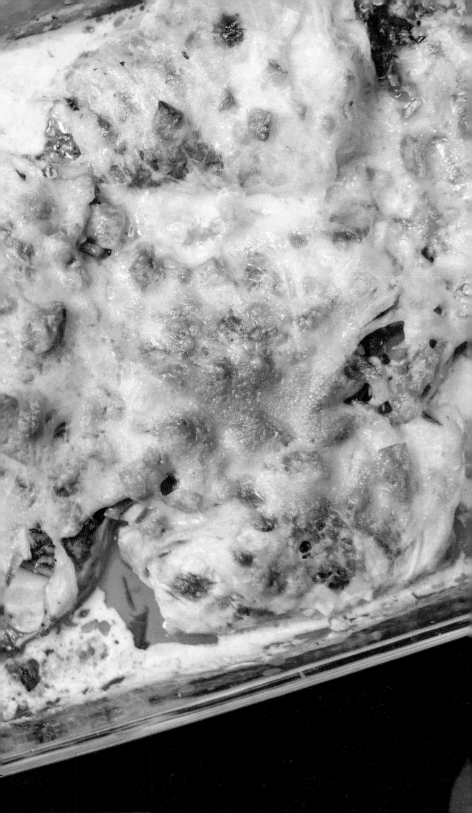

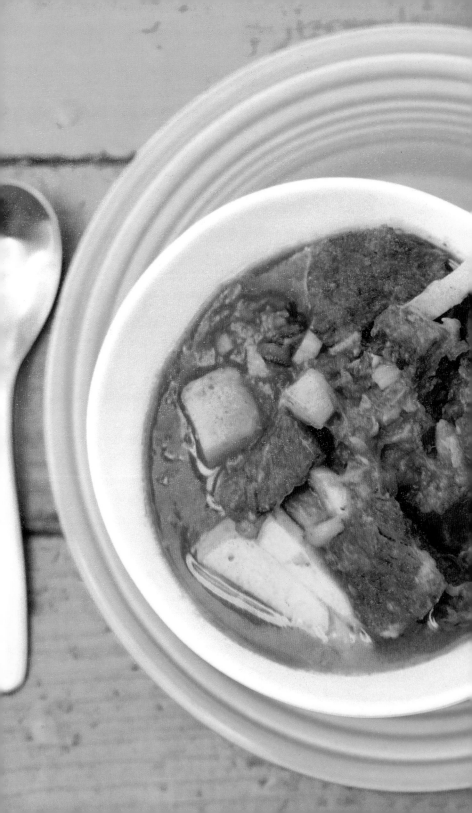

Mexican Stew

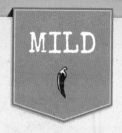

MILD

INGREDIENTS (SERVES 6-8)

- 2 1/2 tablespoons Chili Powder (pg. 17)
- 2 teaspoons sea salt
- 1/2 teaspoon cumin
- 2 lbs grassfed beef stew, cubed
- 1 tablespoon grassfed butter (or other fat source)
- 2 cups onion, chopped
- 1 mild green chile (Anaheim or poblano), chopped
- 5 garlic cloves, minced
- 1/2 cup water
- 1 sweet potato, diced
- 2 cups diced tomatoes
- 1 cup chicken broth
- 1 orange, juiced
- 1 lime, juiced plus more for garnish
- 2 chayote squash, sliced
- fresh cilantro (optional)

DIRECTIONS

01 Combine 1 1/2 tablespoons Chili Powder (pg. 17), sea salt and cumin in a large bowl. Add beef and toss to coat.

02 Heat a Dutch oven or any deep pot over medium heat. After a minute melt butter (or your fat of choice), reduce heat to medium-low, add half the meat and brown on all sides, 5 to 7 minutes. Transfer to a plate and brown the rest of the meat and set aside.

03 Add onions, chiles and garlic to the same pot. Cook, stirring, for 5-7 minutes until onions become translucent.

04 Add an additional 1 tablespoon of chili powder and stir until vegetables are coated.

05 Add water and simmer until most of the liquid has evaporated.

06 Stir in sweet potato, diced tomatos, chicken broth, orange juice, lime juice and reserved beef. Return to a simmer, reduce heat, cover and cook until beef easily separates with the pull of a fork, 1 1/2 to 2 hours.

07 Stir in sliced chayote squash and cook until tender, 10 to 15 minutes.

08 Serve stew in a bowl garnished with lime wedges and fresh cilantro.

Enjoy! :)

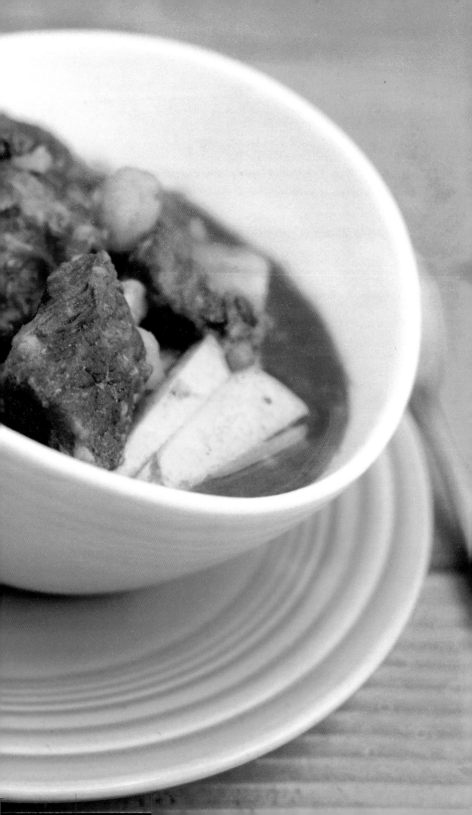

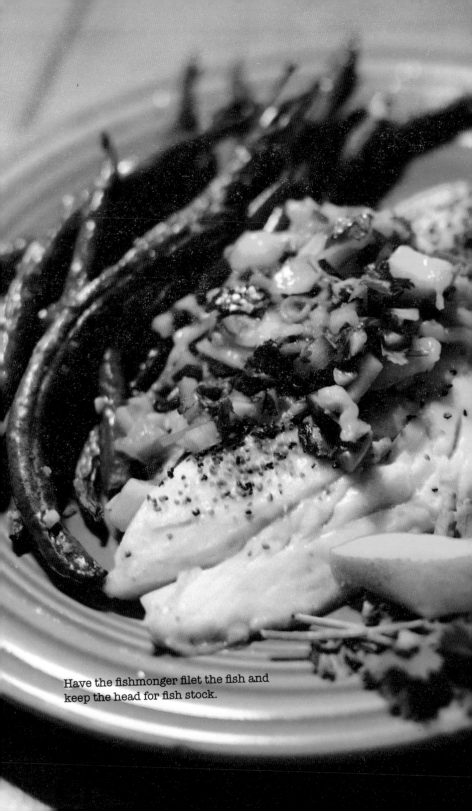

Have the fishmonger filet the fish and
keep the head for fish stock.

Baked Snapper

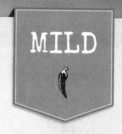

INGREDIENTS (SERVES 2)

1 1/2 lbs fresh wild-caught yellowtail snapper
sea salt, to taste
coarse ground black pepper, to taste

DIRECTIONS

01 Preheat oven to 350 F.

02 Season both sides of the snapper filet with sea salt and black pepper.

03 Lay on a rimmed baking sheet and bake for 12-15 minutes, or until skin flakes with a fork.

04 Remove from oven and let sit 1-2 minutes.

05 Serving with Mango Salsa (pg. 19) and Not the Typical Beans (pg. 49).

Enjoy! :)

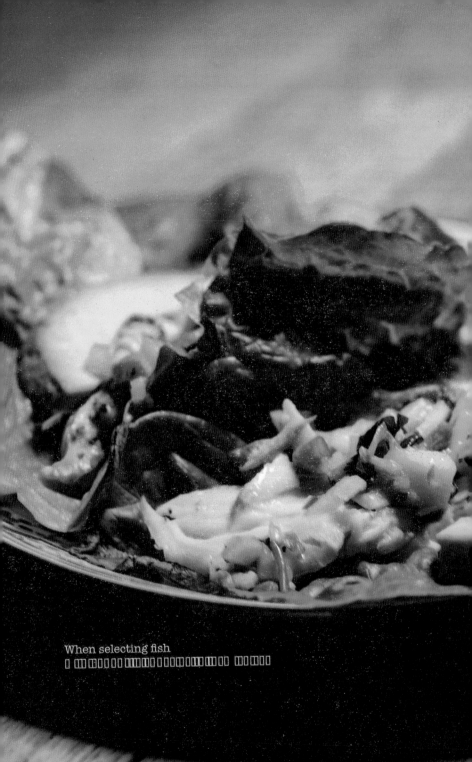

When selecting fish

Fish Tacos with Mango Salsa

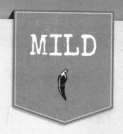

MILD

INGREDIENTS (SERVES 2)

1 1/2 lbs fresh wild-caught fish*
sea salt, to taste
coarse ground black pepper, to taste
1 head romaine lettuce
Mango Salsa (pg. 19)
fresh cilantro (optional)
1-2 limes, quartered (optional)

DIRECTIONS

01 Preheat oven to 350 F.

02 Season both sides of the fish with sea salt and black pepper.

03 Lay on a rimmed baking sheet and bake for 12-15 minutes, or until skin flakes with a fork.

04 Remove from oven and let sit 1-2 minutes while you prepare the taco shells.

05 Carefully separate individual romaine leaves, rinse and pat dry between two paper towels.

06 Transfer two leaves to each plate.

07 Gently shred the fish with a fork and transfer to each romaine leaf. Be aware of the bones.

08 Top with Mango Salsa (pg. 19), fresh cilantro and serve with lime wedges for an extra added drop of citrus.

Enjoy! :)

* I recommend Baked Snapper (pg. 97), though any firm fish such as sea bass, cod, mahi mahi, shrimp or salmon

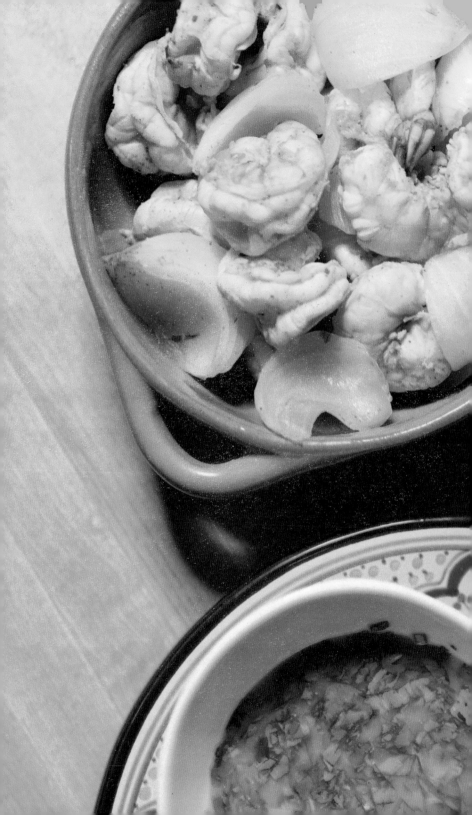

Chile Marinated Shrimp

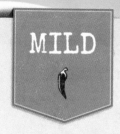

INGREDIENTS (SERVES 2)

1 lb raw peeled & deveined shrimp
1 tablespoon sea salt
4 limes, juiced
1/2 tablespoon Chili Powder (pg. 17)
1 onion, chunked

DIRECTIONS

01 Remove the tails from the shrimp.

02 Add shrimp, sea salt, lime juice and Chili Powder (pg. 17) to a 1 gallon zip lock bag. Seal the bag and mix everything together.

03 Refrigerate for 30 minutes.

04 Saute marinated shrimp and onions over medium heat for 7-9 minutes, or until shrimp turns pink.

05 Serve with Spanish Rice (pg. 45) and use C³: Creamy Coconut Cilantro Dressing (pg. 31) as a dipping sauce.

Enjoy! :)

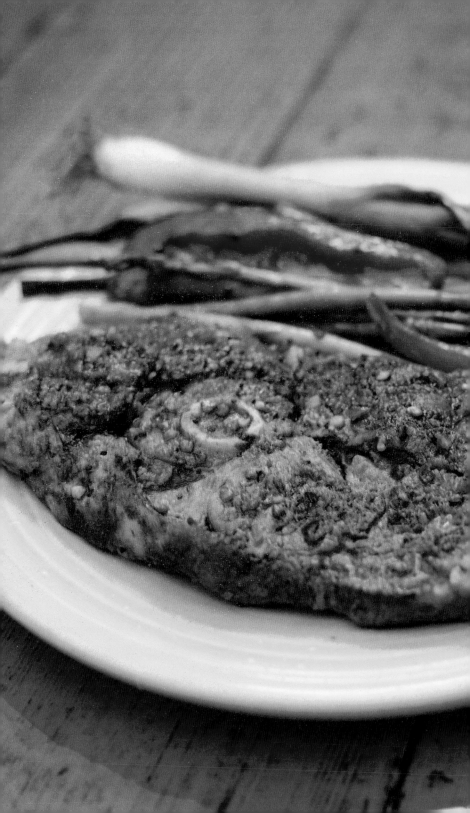

Fire-Rubbed Lamb Steaks

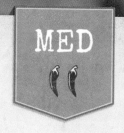

INGREDIENTS (SERVES 2)

- 2 (10 oz) grassfed lamb steaks
- 1/2 teaspoon black pepper
- 1 teaspoon cumin
- 1 teaspoon red pepper flakes
- 5 garlic cloves, minced
- 1 teaspoon sea salt
- 1 teaspoon organic cocoa powder

DIRECTIONS

01 Remove lamb steaks from packaging, transfer to a plate and thaw (if necessary).

02 In a small bowl combine black pepper, cumin, red pepper flakes, garlic cloves, sea salt and cocoa powder to prepare the spice rub. On a clean, flat tray or plate shake the spice rub out evenly.

03 Press both sides of steak into the spice mixture.

04 Heat a grill or grill pan over medium-high heat. If using a grill pan, add one steak at a time and turn down heat so the spices don't burn off. Cook 3-4 minutes per side (for medium) and repeat with second steak.

05 Let meat rest for 1-2 minutes before serving.

06 Serve with grilled vegetables, mild salsa or Dragon Guacamole (pg. 33).

Enjoy! :)

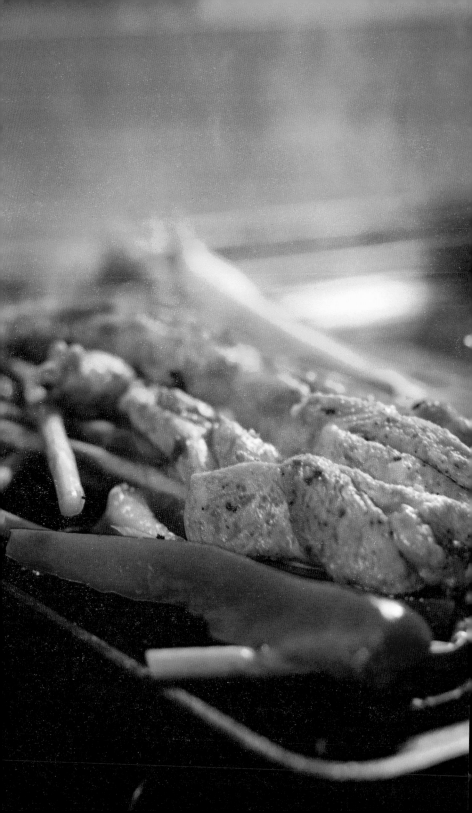

Lemon Chicken Fajitas

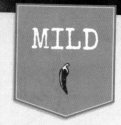

MILD

INGREDIENTS (SERVES 3–4)

- 1-2 tablespoons sea salt
- 1 1/2 teaspoons Chili Powder (pg. 17)
- 1/2 teaspoon red pepper flakes
- 1 lemon, juiced
- 1 tablespoon coconut oil, melted
- 1 1/2 lbs boneless chicken thighs (or breast), cut into strips
- 1 red pepper, sliced
- 1 green pepper, sliced
- 4 green onions, whole
- 1 bunch thin asparagus, trimmed of wooden ends
- 1 teaspoon olive oil

DIRECTIONS

01 Combine 1 tablespoon sea salt, Chili Powder (pg. 17), red pepper, lemon juice, coconut oil and chicken strips in a large bowl. Mix well to coat chicken evenly. Marinate meat in refrigerator for 2-3 hours.

02 Add sliced red and green pepper, green onions and trimmed asparagus to a large bowl. Drizzle in olive oil and sea salt, to taste. Mix well to coat all vegetables.

03 Saute peppers, onion and asparagus until crisp, 1-3 minutes, on a grill or grill pan over medium heat. Transfer to a plate and set aside.

04 Cook chicken over medium-high heat for 5-6 minutes (no pink). Return pepper mixture to pan to warm together.

05 Serve on a tortilla, in a romaine lettuce leaf or as-is.

Enjoy! :)

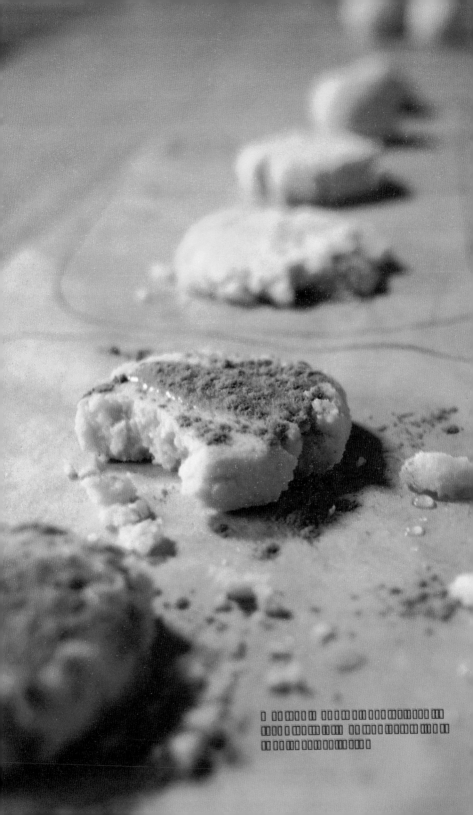

Mexican Sugar Cookies

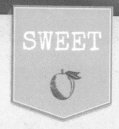

INGREDIENTS (MAKES 25-30 COOKIES)

2 cups blanched almonds
2-3 tablespoons coconut oil, melted
1/4 cup coconut concentrate
1 teaspoon sea salt
raw honey, melted
cinnamon, to taste

DIRECTIONS

01 Preheat oven to 350 F.

02 Add almonds to a food processor and process. Stop the
    blade when almonds line the sides, push the almonds
    down, add some coconut oil and continue to process.
    After 3-5 minutes it will reach an almond butter
    consistency.

03 Add coconut concentrate and sea salt, process until well
    combined.

04 Use a tablespoon to scoop out the batter, roll into balls
    and transfer to a baking stone or rimmed baking sheet.

05 Bake cookies for 7 minutes.

06 Remove from oven and transfer to parchment lined
    counter top. You can keep the cookies in ball form or use
    a wide spatula to flatten them out.

07 Let cookies cool for 1-2 minutes. Serve plain, drizzle with
    raw honey or sprinkle with cinnamon.

08 These cookies are best served immediately (warm) or
    frozen. Freeze leftovers in a sealed container, separated
    by parchment paper so they don't stick.

Enjoy! :)

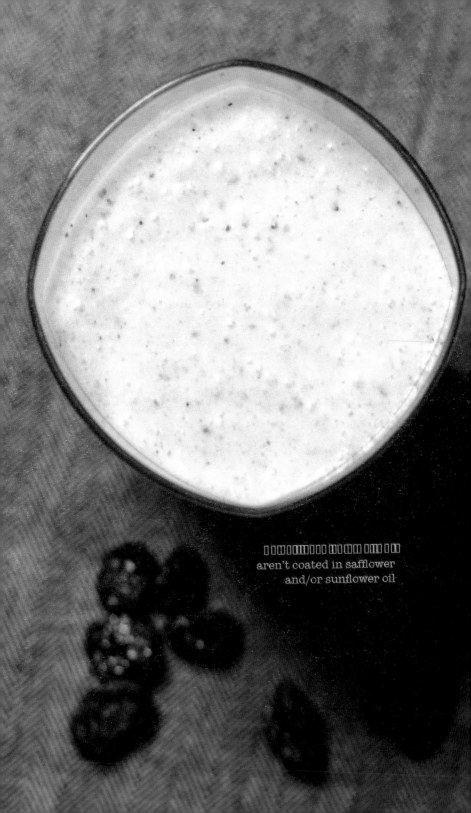

aren't coated in safflower
and/or sunflower oil

Banana Coconut Raisin Smoothie

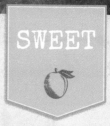

INGREDIENTS (MAKES 2 CUPS)

- 1/2 cup coconut milk
- 2 bananas
- 1/4 cup raisins
- 1/8 cup cacao nibs
- 1-2 cups water
- 3-4 tablespoons coconut concentrate
- 1-2 tablespoons cinnamon
- 1/4 teaspoon nutmeg
- 3-4 ice cubes (optional)

DIRECTIONS

01 Add coconut milk, bananas, raisins, cacao nibs, water, coconut concentrate, cinnamon and nutmeg to a blender. (Add ice for a cold drink).

02 Process until smooth.

03 Pour into glasses and serve.

Enjoy! :)

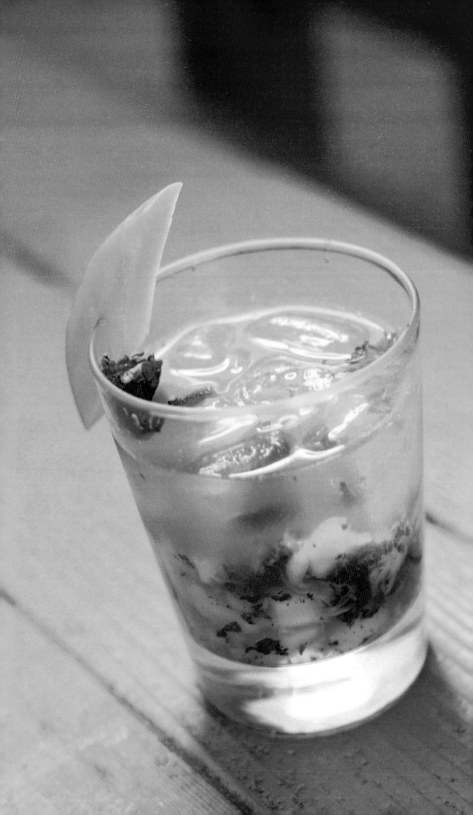

Mango Mojito

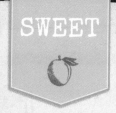

INGREDIENTS (SERVES 1)

1 fresh mint sprig, muddled
1/2 cup mango, cubed and muddled
1 teaspoon raw honey
1/2 lime, juiced
1/2 cup ice
1 1/2 oz 100% agave tequila
2 1/2 oz club soda

DIRECTIONS

01 Muddle the mint and mango with a splash of club soda.

02 Add mint, mango, raw honey and the juice of half of a lime to a highball glass.

03 Add ice, followed by the tequila and club soda.

04 Stir to combine and serve.

Enjoy! :)

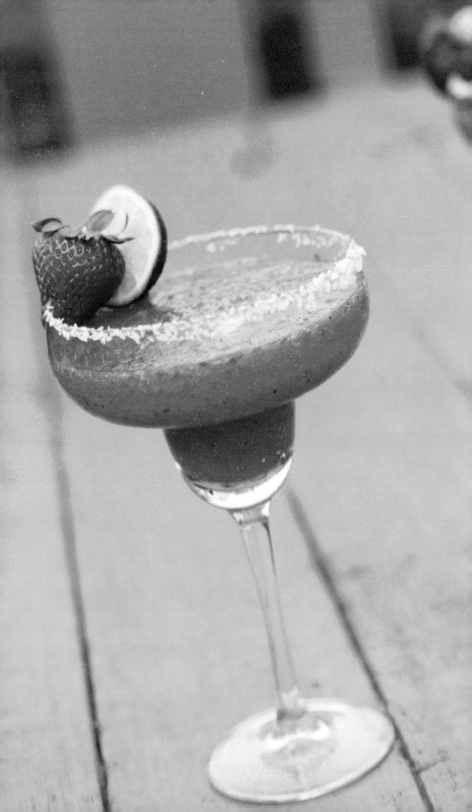

Frozen Strawberry Paleo-rita

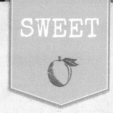

SWEET

INGREDIENTS (SERVES 4)

3 1/2 cups ice
1 1/2 limes, juiced (remaining half used for rim)
3 oz 100% agave tequila
12 oz fresh strawberries, hulled & extra for rim
1 teaspoon raw honey
fine salt, for rim

DIRECTIONS

01 Add ice, lime juice, tequila, strawberries and raw honey
    to a blender.

02 Blend until ice is crushed and ingredients are combined.

03 Pour fine salt out on a small plate, slide a lime half around
    the edge of each glass and dip glass in salt to line the rim.

04 Pour Paleo-rita in each glass.

05 Garnish with a slice of lime and a fresh strawberry and
    serve.

Enjoy! :)

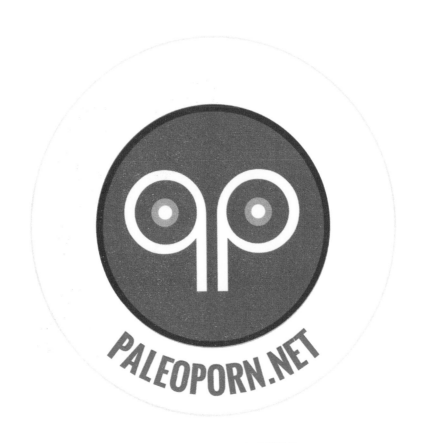

HUNGRY FOR MORE?

Go to PaleoPorn.net to find Marla's ever expanding
library of Paleo Recipes and cookbooks

PIGSKIN PALEO

GAMEDAY PALEO RECIPES
NOT FOR CHEESEHEADS

MARLA SARRIS
FOREWORD BY VIC MAGARY

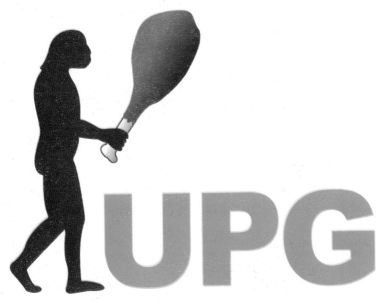

UPG

The Ultimate Guide To The Paleo Diet

UltimatePaleoGuide.com is the #1 resource on the web about the paleo diet – curating paleo food lists, recipes, and meal plans to help you make your transition to the paleo diet as smooth as possible.

For more paleo goodness and your free paleo starter kit, visit Ultimate Paleo Guide.

ENJOY THIS BOOK? LET ME KNOW!

Go to LosPaleo.com/amazon to leave a review
and tweet to me at @MARLAsarris

Thanks!

Made in the USA
Lexington, KY
22 June 2013